PODIATRIC MANAGEMENT
OF THE DIABETIC FOOT

Podiatric Medicine and Surgery

A Monograph Series

Morton D. Fielding, D.P.M., *Managing Editor*

Edward H. Lazo, D.P.M., *Managing Editor*

PODIATRIC MANAGEMENT OF THE DIABETIC FOOT

ROBERT RAKOW, D.P.M., F.A.C.F.S.

Diplomate, American Board of Podiatric Surgery
Attending-in-Charge, Division of Podiatry
Maimonides Medical Center
Chief, Division of Podiatry
Coney Island Hospital
Chief, Division of Podiatry
Caledonian Hospital
Brooklyn, New York

FUTURA PUBLISHING COMPANY
MOUNT KISCO, NEW YORK
1979

This volume is dedicated to my parents
Lena and Abraham

Published by:
Futura Publishing Company
295 Main Street
Mount Kisco, New York 10549

LC: 79-50115
ISBN: 0-87993-119-1

Composition by Topel Typographic Corporation, New York City

Introduction

Since diabetes mellitus is a systemic disease in which the patient is unable to properly metabolize the carbohydrate molecule, its overall management and treatment belong to the internist. However, the total care of the diabetic patient encompasses many fields and requires a multidisciplinary approach. As part of the health care team, the podiatrist treats the diabetic foot. This text is written to serve as a practical guide for the podiatrist who endeavors to deal with the diabetic foot. He must not only be able to recognize and treat the local foot pathology to which the diabetic is heir, he must also understand the basic methods and rationale necessary to control the diabetic state.

While this book will cover the prudent podiatric management of the diabetic foot, it is never inferred that the podiatrist is to assume responsibility for the overall management of the diabetic patient. The material set forth in this work is gleaned from 35 years of practical experience in caring for the feet of diabetic patients. In the chapters that follow, I will discuss the use of insulin in various clinical stages of preoperative, operative and postoperative care. Proper insulin coverage is vital. The internist has various types of insulin at his disposal in the management of the patient. I shall not touch upon the use of oral agents. The co-admitting physician should be conversant with techniques used to control hyperglycemia and ketonuria if either or both are present. Some drugs used by the podiatrist may alter the glucose level. The podiatrist should alert the physician, who should then act accordingly.

The longevity and lifestyle of the diabetic have markedly improved with the advent of insulin. However, the danger of complications is ever present — notably retinopathy, neuropathy and vascular degenerative changes. I will not discuss academic philosophy or sophistication of complications in detail, but will, rather, attempt to describe the management of these complications when they do occur. The chapters of this book can be read in any order, depending upon the experience of the reader. The novice should read it as written. The podiatrist experienced in treating diabetics can use it as a reference guide to update or renew details as needed.

Vascular disease and neuropathy play major roles in the clinical picture to be studied. The patient who has a neuropathic foot suffers from impaired sensation. Neuropathic ulcers are common lesions that the podiatrist sees as a result of diabetes. Retinopathy impairs vision and makes self foot care dangerous. The patient who has diabetes should never treat his own feet. A non-diabetic member of the family can help in only one way, and that is by testing the temperature of the bath water. Diabetics with peripheral neuropathy do not feel the parameters of hot and cold. It is not uncommon to find thermal gangrene in these people. Diabetics should bathe only in tepid water tested by a non-diabetic person. Just as a patient who suffers from diabetic neuropathy does not feel the extremes in temperature, so a patient with poor vascularity cannot dissipate the heat normally; hence, thermal gangrene.

The podiatrist who undertakes the treatment and care of the diabetic foot takes on a unique responsibility. He is handling a foot that is vulnerable to infection. He is handling a foot that is vulnerable to gangrene. At the present time, every diabetic clinic throughout the United States has a podiatrist on service. These centers recognize the podiatrist's role in lowering the amputation rate in the diabetic patient. In spite of meticulous care, there will always be that patient whose limb is beyond redemption. Life and death situations are possible in treating diabetic feet. Minor trauma or minor infection can trigger a sequence of events resulting in the death of a patient. I have seen a superficial paronychia end in catastrophe.

Even as medical care becomes more specialized, it remains true that most often the one who routinely looks at the feet of the patient is the podiatrist. It is incumbent upon him to recognize lesions in the pre-gangrenous state. The podiatrist who cares for the diabetic foot cannot do so alone. He needs the aid of the internist, the vascular surgeon and a well equipped hospital. He needs to be part of the interdisciplinary team approach to the diabetic patient.

INTRODUCTION

This text will describe the management of feet afflicted with macrovascular and microvascular disease. In macrovascular disease pedal pulses are diminished or absent; however, one should not be lulled into a false sense of security if a pedal pulse is present. This is not an indication that the patient is free from danger at the distal end of the toe. Here minute vessels can be easily occluded by trauma, such as the touch of a finger, the pressure of a shoe, or spontaneous infarct leading to gangrene. Spontaneous infarction is the most common cause of gangrene in the diabetic patient. It is caused by small vessel disease and not by outside influences such as shoe pressure or iatrogenic causes. Gangrene can develop in a digit despite meticulous care. Exquisite control of blood sugar is not tantamount to a life free of diabetic complications. Through the years, I have seen minutely monitored and minutely altered blood glucose in patients who, nevertheless, have developed vascular changes that resulted in skin lesions and necrosis.

The podiatrist who treats the diabetic foot must be well schooled in all the medical disciplines by keeping abreast of the latest techniques in diagnosis, management and therapy. For the past 30 years I have been proposing, and teaching my students, this basic tenet: *Please treat our patients with the maximum of care, the maximum of tenderness and a minimum of trauma!* I have found no phase of podiatry more fulfilling than that aspect which concerns itself with the care of the diabetic foot.

Editor's Foreword

The management of the diabetic foot is a very important part of most podiatrists' daily practice. When Dr. Rakow offered to share his 35 years of experience and expertise, we were thrilled. Here was an opportunity to formally present the current "state of the art" to the profession. Although a team approach is strongly advised, this book provides the student podiatrist and the seasoned practitioner with sound management techniques and philosophy for contemporary podiatric practice in dealing with the diabetic patient's foot condition.

The dramatic results of Dr. Rakow's methods will speak for themselves. The positive impact of podiatry on the diabetic population is formidable, with maintenance care being just as important as the life and limb saving procedures described herein. We are cautious not to take careful and considerate conservative care for granted. With this book, we offer to pass the torch of knowledge and experience to the novice and to rekindle the light of affirmation to the practicing Doctor of Podiatric Medicine. This text is produced by a podiatrist who sincerely cares for his fellow practitioners and for their (our) patients.

Edward H. Lazo, D.P.M., F.A.C.F.S.

Contents

CHAPTER 1

History and Examination of the Foot

PROPER HISTORY

The history of the diabetic patient is important, if not vital, to the podiatrist caring for the diabetic foot. At the outset, I should like to call to the podiatrist's attention the fact that the patient may or may not be a good historian. The patient all too often willfully lies with regard to his history. If possible, the entire history should be confirmed by another member of the family.

The obvious essentials, such as name, age, marital status, address and next of kin, need no comment. The salient features of the diabetic's history are:

(1) the duration of the patient's diabetes (length of time that he or she is a known diabetic);

(2) the date and place of the last blood sugar determination;

(3) the date and place of the last urinalysis;

(4) the name and address of the physician who is managing the patient's diabetes;

(5) the date of the most recent visit to his physician;

(6) the type and amount of insulin or oral agents he is taking;

(7) the name and address of any previous podiatrist consulted by the patient;

(8) the type and frequency of foot care received elsewhere.

Personal hygiene, foot gear and personal habits (e.g., smoking) should be noted. Whether the patient usually walks barefooted about his home is as important to note as is whether or not the patient cuts his or her own toe nails, and whether he or she has ever been known to use corn plasters, pumice stone or other home remedies as a substitute for professional care. It is important to know if the patient has any known drug allergies, specifically if the patient has had allergic reactions to any antibiotics or local anesthetics. It is vital to know if the patient has had insulin reactions (hypoglycemia), and at what time they occur. If the patient gives a history of mid-day reactions and the podiatrist is treating the patient at noon, he should be on alert for signs of hypoglycemia.

In addition, knowledge of any previous foot surgery is imperative. The postoperative course would then be an essential part of the patient's history.

The presence of intermittent claudication and/or nocturnal claudication is essential, as is the walking time and distance. If possible, one should establish the presence of neuropathy. Does the patient feel the difference between grades of temperature? Does he know hot from cold? Does he have paresthesias? Are his toes ever numb? Are his subjective symptoms unilateral or bilateral? The answers to these questions are essential for the proper evaluation of the patient, which the history should provide. The podiatrist must know of any and all medications the patient is taking, including the dosage. Before evaluating the patient, and before any attempt to treat him, the podiatrist should be made aware of any other constitutional disease that the patient has had or does have. The following systemic diseases or syndromes — namely, neurologic disorders, like syringomyelia (paresthesia), petit mal or grand mal seizures; metabolic disorders, such as thyroid or pituitary dysfunctions (osseous deformity); hematologic disorders like Von Willebrand's disease (inability to clot), thrombocytosis, intravascular thrombi or anemia; cardiac disease with resultant peripheral edema; and renal disease (Kimmelstiel-Wilson Disease) — are important in evaluating the diabetic foot.

If a proper history is taken, and I have outlined the essential elements, the podiatrist will be in a much better position to treat his patient. Indeed, he will become a member of the health team.

VASCULAR EXAMINATION OF THE FOOT

Anatomy of the Arterial Pathway of the Lower Extremity

The podiatrist cannot conduct a vascular examination of the

foot without a knowledge of the normal arterial sypply. Therefore, I will outline the arterial tree of the lower extremity.

The femoral artery is the continuation of the external iliac artery. It perforates the inguinal ligament and lies superficially in the femoral triangle. At the apex of the triangle, it passes deep to the sartorius muscle, enters Hunter's canal, and is placed deeply here. At the base of the femoral triangle (Scarpa's triangle), the femoral nerve lies lateral to the artery and the femoral vein lies medial to it. The saphenous nerve enters the subsartorial canal with the femoral artery and runs first on its lateral side, then anterior to it, and finally on its medial side. The femoral artery gives off five branches, namely, the superficial branch which further divides into the circumflex iliac, epigastric and the external pudendal. The other branches of the femoral are the muscular, external pudendal, the descending genicular and the profunda. The femoral artery has a lumen of 0.5 cm at its origin.

The popliteal artery is the direct extension of the femoral. It has a lumen measuring 0.36 cm at the proximal end of the popliteal space. The popliteal artery passes on the medial side of the popliteal fossa, under the semimembranous muscle, and ends at the distal border of the popliteus muscle. At the level of the tibial tubercle, it divides into the anterior and posterior tibial arteries. The posterior tibial artery is the larger of the two terminal branches of the popliteal. The posterior tibial artery has a lumen diameter of 0.28 cm and the anterior tibial has a lumen diameter of 0.21 cm.

The posterior tibial artery runs downward and medially in the posterior aspect of the leg, between the superficial and deep layers of muscle. It passes behind the medial malleolus, where it can be readily palpated. At this point the artery is superior to the posterior tibial nerve and inferior to the saphenous vein. At the level of the medial malleolus, the tendon of the tibialis posticus and the tendon of the flexor digitorum longus lie superficial to the posterior artery, and the tendon of the flexor hallucis longus lies laterally and deeper. The posterior tibial artery is accompanied by two venae comitantes.

The posterior tibial artery gives off several branches. The most important to the podiatrist is the peroneal artery. It has a lumen diameter of 0.12 cm at its origin, which is about 25 mm (1 inch) below the distal border of the popliteus muscle. This artery is very important when one realizes that this vessel is relatively free of occlusive vascular disease.[1] About one inch proximal to the ankle joint it gives off a perforating branch, then passes behind the inferior tibiofibular joint and the lateral malleolus to the lateral side of the heel and foot. It supplies the ankle, the inferior tibiofibular and talocalcaneal joints, and anastomoses with a calcaneal branch of the lateral plantar artery, the tarsal and arcuate branches of the dorsalis pedis artery. The medial and lateral plantar arteries are the terminal branches of the posterior tibial artery. They arise beneath the flexor retinaculum midway between the tip of the medial malleolus and the most prominent aspect of the medial side of the heel. The medial plantar artery is smaller than the lateral plantar artery. The lumen measures approximately 0.03 cm. It passes forward on the medial side of the medial plantar nerve beneath the abductor hallucis and superior to the flexor brevis digitorum. It then travels distally to the head of the first metatarsal bone, where it ends by uniting with the digital branch of the first plantar metatarsal artery, which supplies the medial side of the hallux. In its course distally, it supplies the abductor hallucis and sends branches to adjacent muscles, articulations and the skin. It also gives off three digital branches which anastomose at the base of the three medial interdigital clefts and the medial plantar metatarsal arteries. Some of the cutaneous branches of the medial plantar artery anastomose with the cutaneous branches of the dorsalis pedis artery on the medial aspect of the foot.

The lateral plantar artery, the larger of the two terminal branches of the posterior tibial artery, runs obliquely forward across the plantar aspect of the foot on the lateral side of the lateral plantar nerve. At first, it passes between the flexor brevis digitorum superficially and the flexor accessorius deeply. As it travels laterally, it passes between the flexor brevis digitorum and the abductor minimi digiti. It travels to the medial side of the base of the fifth metatarsal bone. At the base of the fifth metatarsal bone, the lateral plantar artery turns rather abruptly medially and becomes deeper, passing across the bases of the metatarsal bones and the origins of the interossei superficial to the oblique head of the abductor hallucis, to the lateral side of the first metatarsal bone where it anastomoses with the dorsalis pedis artery. The latter part of the lateral plantar artery, passing convexly, forms the plantar arch as it joins the dorsalis pedis artery. The lateral plantar artery, as it crosses from the area of the fifth metatarsal base, gives off four metatarsal branches, which in turn bifurcate to supply the plantar aspect of the fifth, fourth, third, and lateral half of the second toes. Between the base of the fifth metatarsal bone and the first interosseous space, it forms the plantar arch. In addition to the four plantar arteries, it gives off three perforating branches to the dorsal metatarsal arteries and twigs to the tarsal joints and muscles in the area. The plantar aspect and dorsal aspect of the foot have communicating arteries. The first plantar metatarsal artery is a branch of the dorsalis pedis. When the dorsalis pedis dips plantarly to join the lateral plantar artery completing the plantar arch, it gives off the first plantar metatarsal artery.

The medial plantar artery may be very small or absent. When this occurs, its place is taken by branches of the dorsalis pedis or lateral plantar arteries. The lateral plantar artery may also be small or absent. If this should occur, the plantar arch is then formed entirely by the dorsalis pedis.

The anterior tibial artery, as noted previously, is the smaller of the two branches of the popliteal. This vessel originates at the distal border of the popliteus muscle in the back of the leg, passes forward between two slips of the proximal part of the tibialis posterior muscle, and passes through an aperture in the proximal end of the interosseous membrane. As it progresses downward and distally it rests on the anterior surface of the interosseous membrane. Its proximal third lies between the extensor longus digitorum laterally and the tibialis anticus medially. Its middle third lies between the extensor longus hallucis and the tibial anticus. In the distal third of its course, the extensor longus hallucis crosses in front of it and we now have the extensor longus hallucis tendon on the medial aspect and the medial tendon of the extensor longus digitorum on the lateral side. At the ankle, the anterior tibial nerve lies between the anterior tibial artery and the most medial tendon of the extensor longus digitorum.

The dorsalis pedis artery is the direct continuation of the anterior tibial artery. It starts on the anterior aspect of the ankle and runs to the proximal end of the first interosseous space, at which point it gives off the first dorsal metatarsal artery and then passes to the plantar aspect of the foot between the two heads of the first dorsal interosseous muscle to join the lateral plantar artery, thus forming the plantar arch. Superficially, it is covered by skin and fascia. Just before it reaches the first interosseous space, it is crossed by the tendon of the extensor brevis hallucis. It rests upon the head of the talus, the navicular, and the middle cuneiform bones.

The dorsalis pedis sends out cutaneous branches which are distributed to the skin on the dorsum and the medial side of the foot. They also anastomose with branches of the medial plantar artery. Another branch of the dorsalis pedis is the tarsal artery. This branch runs beneath the extensor digitorum brevis, supplying that muscle and all the tarsal joints. It also anastomoses with the perforating branches of the peroneal artery, arcuate and lateral plantar arteries.

Another branch of the dorsalis pedis is the arcuate artery, arising at the medial cuneiform bone. It runs laterally at the bases of the metatarsal bones beneath the long and short extensor tendons. It anastomoses with branches of the tarsal and lateral plantar arteries. It gives off three dorsal metatarsal arteries. These vessels pass through the second, third and fourth interosseous spaces, resting on the interosseus muscles of the three lateral interosseous spaces. They pass to the clefts of the toes, where they divide into two dorsal digital arteries for the adjacent sides of the toes. The lateral side of the fifth toe is supplied by a branch of the most lateral dorsal metatarsal artery. Each dorsal metatarsal artery gives off a posterior perforating branch, which passes through the posterior part of the intermetatarsal space, between the heads of the dorsal interosseous muscle, and anastomoses with the plantar arch and an anterior perforating branch which passes through the anterior part of the space to anastomose with the corresponding plantar metatarsal artery. The first dorsal metatarsal artery arises from the dorsalis pedis and runs distally in the first metatarsal interspace on the dorsal surface of the first dorsal interosseous muscle. It divides into two branches supplying adjacent sides of the hallux and second toes. Just prior to its division, it gives off an artery, the dorsal digital, which passes beneath the tendon of the extensor longus hallucis and supplies the medial aspect of the great toe.

When the dorsalis pedis unites with the lateral plantar artery to complete the plantar arch, it gives rise to the first plantar metatarsal artery. This vessel passes forward in the first metatarsal interspace to the web space, where it divides into plantar digital arteries supplying the adjacent sides of the first and second toes.

Just prior to its division, it gives rise to a plantar digital artery, which in turn supplies the medial aspect of the great toe.[2]

The entire anterior tibial artery may be absent. In such cases, the posterior tibial and peroneal arteries take over.

Physiology of the Arterial Pathway

One must pause and reflect. The arterial tree is not only composed of major vessels. All arteries anastomose with other vessels. The anterior with the posterior, the lateral with the medial, the dorsal with the plantar, thereby forming a complex mechanism for the perfusion of the lower extremity. By studying the arterial anatomy with its vast interchanges, the podiatrist can appreciate the need for watchful waiting. The heel, for example, is supplied by branches of the lateral plantar, posterior tibial and peroneal arteries. There are tiny anastomoses that have lumen diameters in the order of 0.03 cm.

If it were not for this vast network of arteries and arterioles, the upright human would suffer from ischemia to the plantar aspect of the foot. Here one must never lose sight of the fact that an intact sympathetic nervous system with intact nerve supply to the vasa nervorum plays a major role in keeping the plantar aspect of the foot from pressure necrosis.

The distal aspects of the foot and the toes have a double arterial supply, the plantar and the dorsal apparatus. In the main, the plantar metatarsal arteries, arising from the lateral plantar artery, supply the plantar aspect. The dorsum of the foot and toes are supplied by the arcuate, which in turn arises from the dorsalis pedis. There are dorsal metatarsal arteries which complement the plantar arteries supplying the distal ends of the toes. In the event of a loss of the dorsal supply due to occlusion from thrombi or emboli, the foot can be saved if the plantar arterial tree is intact.

One cannot practice podiatry as it concerns the diabetic without having the academic knowledge of the arterial wall. From the femoral artery, indeed, from the aorta to the capillary as we move peripherally, the arterial wall changes from a highly elastic tube to structures with less elasticity and contractile abilities. The femoral artery is an example of a highly elastic vessel, the dorsalis pedis is an example of a moderately contractile vessel, and the millions of arterioles are examples of highly contractile structures. These microscopic vessels capable of varying the diameter of the lumen are responsible for the blood supply to the local areas.

The podiatrist caring for the diabetic foot should be aware of the fact that the very essence of tissue viability, in the final analysis, is determined at the level of the arterioles and capillaries. When we consider the adventitia, clearly defined in medium-sized arteries such as the popliteal and posterior tibial, we find this layer to be rich in networks of collagen and elastic fibers. As we progress to the arterioles, we find a marked reduction in elastic and collagenic material. Conversely, the microscopic arterioles, other than having an endothelial lining, have a wall proportionally larger in smooth muscle than the "parent" vessel, the femoral. Actually, the ratio of lumen size to wall thickness is greater in the arterioles than in large lumen vessels (0.67 in arterioles, compared to 0.25 in larger vessels). Smooth muscle contraction is more effective in changing vessel tension and elasticity than in controlling blood flow.

One cannot be a student of the vascular tree without an academic knowledge of the vasa vasorum. We are aware of the fact that the blood vessels carry nutrients for maintaining the viability of tissue. But, what of the viability of the vessels themselves? It is in this context that the vasa vasorum plays a most important role. Nourishment of the inner layers of the vessel wall is derived from the flow of blood through the lumen. The products necessary for survival pass through the endothelial layer and into the cells beyond for a distance of 0.35–0.5 mm.[3] Arteries having a wall thickness greater than 0.35 mm must have a mechanism to penetrate the adventitia and media. This feat is accomplished by the vasa vasorum. This arterial supply never communicates with the lumen of the vessel. It originates from branches of the artery which return to penetrate the artery's own adventitia. There is a complete network of minute vessels in a circumferential pattern in the vessel wall. They empty into a huge network of venules. Vessels having a lumen of 1 mm or less do not have vasa vasorum. Arterioles, therefore, have no vasa vasorum. They do, however, possess a band of smooth muscle which controls the size of the lumen prior to the formation of the capillary. Capillaries consist only of a layer of endothelial cells and a basement membrane enclosed by a sheath of connective tissue. Unlike the arterioles they do not have contractile apparatus. The size of their lumen is governed by external intracellar pressure.

Hemodynamics of the Arterial Tree

The same volume of blood which enters the lower extremity at the inguinal ligament reaches the entire area of the foot. The lumen size as we progress distally from the femoral artery becomes smaller. In fact, in the area of the toes, the vessels are microscopic in size. The bifurcation of a vessel increases the velocity of the blood flow. It must be understood, however, that bifurcation is not the modus operandi for increasing velocity of blood flow. When a vessel gives off side branches, each branch has a smaller lumen than the parent vessel. Collectively there is a marked increase in cross-sectional area and an increase in velocity of blood flow.[1]

Atherosclerosis Obliterans

I have outlined the normal vascular supply of the foot. It is common knowledge that the diabetic is subject to early and extensive organic occlusion of any artery or group of arteries. Severe ischemia may result in gangrene in the extremity or loss of life. I have found that only when an occlusion develops more rapidly than collateral circulation does tissue die. If the blood flow is less than that required at rest, infarction and death of tissue results.

Vasospasm

The vasospastic syndrome, as described by Raynaud in 1862, primarily affects the upper extremity. The toes have been known to be affected. Therefore, it is important for the podiatrist to be familiar with the disease. This section of the text is devoted to the recognition of pathology that affects the blood flow to the foot.

The patient with vasospastic disease has intermittent subjective complaints. Objective signs are likewise intermittent and sporadic. As opposed to the arteriosclerotic, these patients are usually young, and females are more often affected. The seizure is usually precipitated by exposure to cold. Emotions, however, can exacerbate the clinical picture.

A clinical episode of Raynaud's Disease can commence as Raynaud's phenomena. The characteristic picture is a pale distal end of the toe which gradually progresses proximally as the vasoconstriction persists. This picture is followed by cyanosis of the toe. During the entire episode, which may last thirty to sixty minutes, the pedal pulses remain palpable. The patient will complain of numbness and paresthesia of the part or parts affected. Differentiation of vasospastic and organic occlusive disease will be discussed later in the text at the appropriate sequence.

The vascular examination of the foot is initially carried out by inspection and palpation. The vascular tree, as I have pointed out previously, is a maze of interconnecting, communicating vessels. The capillaries are one-layered microscopic tubes of endothelium whose wall acts as a semi-permeable membrane, which, in the final analysis, is the mechanism which maintains viability of tissues.

PHYSICAL EXAMINATION OF THE FOOT

Inspection

The color and temperature of the skin can be factors in determining the adequacy of the blood flow to the foot. The following observations and conclusions are useful to the podiatrist in determining patency and perfusion of the skin of the foot:

(a) The skin of the foot with normal vascularity appears pale pink and is warm.

(b) Cold pale skin is a sign of restricted blood flow.

(c) Cyanotic appearance of the skin is indicative of a poor blood flow. The degree of cyanosis can be directly proportional to the degree of arteriosclerotic disease.

(d) The appearance of a cold, red inflammatory reaction at the site of an infection is an indication of poor blood flow. The prognosis, therefore, is considered grave.[4] The podiatrist must train himself to detect differences in skin temperature. An experienced observer can detect degrees of gradations in the order of 1° to 2°F. If the examining podiatrist observes either a redness of tissue or a pallor of tissue, he should be able to detect variations in skin temperature. If the inflammatory process is unilateral, the objective observation is simple. The podiatrist should gently run his palms from the mid-leg area distally to the toes. Again, if there are temperature changes, they are readily noted.

The appearance of the skin is often a clue to the presence of an undiagnosed diabetic. The callus tissue appears macerated in the absence of hyperdrosis. The diabetic will frequently develop calluses which are soft in texture, but, extensive in character.

The interdigital spaces are frequently the source of mycotic and yeast (monilia) infections. The treatment will depend on the etiology. It is, therefore, necessary to establish the causative agent. Figure 1 is a KOH preparation of the skin of a diabetic, interdigital epithelium. The typical hyphae are shown in the center. This is characteristic of Trichophyton rubrum. Figure 2 is a KOH preparation of the interdigital yeast infestation. The typical pseudohyphae and budding of the Candida is seen in the center of the microphotograph.

Skin Disorders

There are no specific characteristics pathognomonic of the diabetic with nail changes. The diabetic is heir to the usual changes seen in the non-diabetic. Onychogryphosis, onychauxis and dystrophic nails are seen with the same frequency in the diabetic and non-diabetic. The one glaring exception is chronic, recurrent paronychia. When this condition occurs without apparent cause, the podiatrist must rule in or rule out diabetes mellitus. If the diabetic patient has an impairment in blood flow, nutritional changes may occur in skin, nail and hair growth. If there is an obstruction in blood flow, the nails may become brittle, discolored and ridged. Clinically, one must rule out mycotic invasion of the nail. The presence or absence of hair is a very unreliable test for vascularity. I have seen hair growing on the dorsum of toes and frank gangrene present proximal to the hair site. More reliable is the presence of hair on one limb. Unilateral hair growth may be a sign of occlusive vascular disease of the limb free of hair. It is wise to ask the patient if and when he had hair growth on an extremity prior to making a clinical judgment. Premonitory evidences of gangrene in the diabetic foot are vesicles, hemorrhagic blebs and bullae. Sudden onset of coldness, pain and mottled skin is a sign of acute arterial obstruction. This is usually the result of an embolus or, more rarely, thrombus formation in a major blood vessel. The

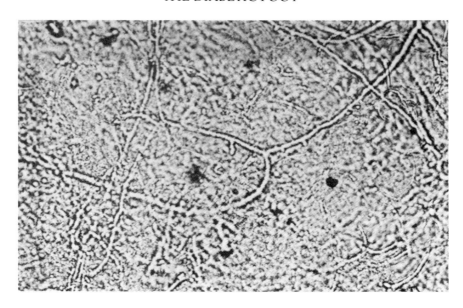

Figure 1. Typical potassium hydroxide preparation of the skin showing the hyphae of a dermatophyte (Trichophyton rubrum).

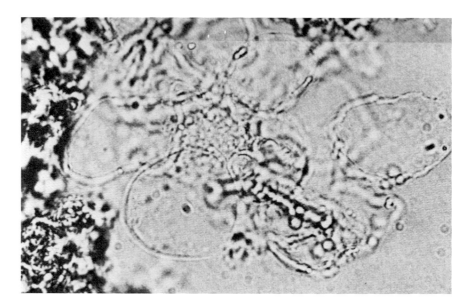

Figure 2. KOH preparation of skin lesion showing pseudohyphae. These are budding yeast cells (Candida).

examiner's fingers and hand are the most important instruments in attempting to evaluate the peripheral blood flow. He needs only to recognize this fact and train himself. I have mentioned the necessity for inspecting variations in skin temperature. There is no instrument more sensitive than the experienced clinician's fingers. The podiatrist should be aware of the fact that the temperature of the skin of the toes is approximately ten to fifteen degrees below body temperature.[5] By simply passing one's hand gently down the leg to the toes, one can detect the sudden drop in temperature at the level of arterial obstruction. Skin having normal perfusion is warm. Poorly vascularized skin is cool or cold.

A test frequently used to determine adequate blood flow is momentary pressure of the finger to the distal end of a toe. If the return to normal color is achieved it is considered to be indicative of normal blood flow. This test is inaccurate and fraught with danger. It has no place in the armamentarium of diagnostic aids. The temperature of the toes is important. If the toes are cold and red (rubor), blanch on pressure, and quickly return to the previous "red" state, they must be considered to be poorly nourished. On the other hand, a cold pale toe can be made lighter in color by the pressure of an examining finger. The return of color will be slow due to constriction, not occlusion, of minute vessels in the skin. This observation is not to be interpreted as a sign of circulatory deficiency. It is wise to elevate the foot. Apply digital pressure to the distal end of the toe and observe color changes.

Venous Filling Time

The following is a reliable test to ascertain blood flow to the foot. It is as reliable as any instrument or device known in establishing the efficiency of the peripheral blood flow. The test is performed as follows:

Place the patient on his back. Elevate both extremities above the level of the heart. Observe until the veins on the dorsum of the foot collapse completely. This is due to the fact that the blood in the venocapillary bed empties into the systemic circulation while the peripheral arterial pressure is so low and the rate of arterial flow so slow in the diseased extremity that these veins remain collapsed. Now, when the patient is quickly placed in the sitting position with the extremities lowered, an accurate record is taken of the time that it takes for the veins on the dorsum of the foot to fill with blood. Since competent lunar valves in the venous tree of the extremity prevent a regurgitation of blood into these dorsal veins, it is obvious that the only way in which these veins can fill is with blood which has passed from the arterial pathways through the capillaries of the foot. It is easily comprehensible that the more profound the obstruction to the arterial flow, the slower will be the rate of the filling of the veins on the dorsum of the foot. In a limb with a normal arterial flow, the collapsed veins will take less than ten seconds to fill. Where it takes more than ten seconds for these veins to show evidence of filling, one may suspect obstruction to arterial flow. I have found that in cases with the severest degrees of obstruction, such as after femoral or popliteal artery thrombosis and where practically no collateral flow is present, the venous filling time may be as great as ninety seconds. It should be noted that the presence of varicose veins in a leg does not affect the accuracy of this test. The valves at the ankle are always competent, even with the most bulbous varicose veins of the leg.

If the patient has unilateral occlusive vascular disease, which is often the case, the results of this test are dramatic. The limb with normal flow will show filling of the dorsal veins within ten seconds. The contralateral limb with occlusive vascular disease will fill in thirty or more seconds. Allow the patient to remain seated with his feet in the dependent position for two to three minutes. The foot with poor blood supply will be cyanotic. In bilateral occlusive vascular disease the veins on the dorsum may take a minute to fill and both limbs are cyanotic in the dependent position.

Skin Turgor

When the arterial flow to a limb becomes interrupted, filtration pressure drops distal to the obstruction. As a result, the filtration pressure in the capillaries supplied by the involved artery becomes affected, and thus directly influences the mechanism of metabolic exchange through the capillary wall. One of the specific effects of this disturbance is a reduction in the amount of water and electrolyte passing through the capillary wall into the circulation, which is recognized clinically as loss of turgor. It can be seen readily by the very simple technique of pulling up a fold of skin and studying the rate at which the skin returns to its normal resting position on release. Normally the skin is so elastic that it returns to its resting position immediately after stretching, just like a new rubber band. The skin of dehydrated tissue, however, has a tendency to delay this return, comparable with the inelastic properties of an old rubber band. In patients with unilateral occlusive vascular disease, either from embolus or thrombosis, the difference in skin turgor is striking. The onset of embolic vascular occlusion is sudden and acute. The clinical picture clearly is impending catastrophe.

Palpation of Pedal Pulses

The dorsalis pedis and posterior tibial pulses are readily palpable in the foot with normal blood supply. The dorsalis pedis is felt on the dorsal aspect of the foot at the level of the navicular and the head of the talus. It is best detected lateral to the tendon of the extensor longus hallucis at this level. The posterior tibial artery can be palpated just lateral and posterior to the medial malleolus. When attempting to palpate the dorsalis pedis, it is wise to hold the calcaneus firm while the foot is in slight dorsiflexion. The posterior tibial pulse can also be felt at this site; however, the foot should be in slight plantar flexion. The posterior tibial pulse may not be felt in the obese foot or the foot that is edematous. It must be kept in mind that the foot may have a normal blood flow and have non-palpable pulses. Collens and Wilensky reported the dorsalis pedis pulsation may not be palpable in up to 19% of feet with no occlusive vascular disease.[5] The posterior tibial pulse may be absent bilaterally in 1% of the normal adult population. The student of peripheral vascular disease must realize that no one indicator can rule in or rule out vascular disease. Only the assessment of the total picture can give the astute podiatrist a yard stick in ascertaining the adequacy of the arterial flow to the foot. In a series of 201 reported cases, Rakow and Friedman[6] found that 80% of the patients examined (160 patients) had pulseless feet, and 90% of these patients had dystrophic nails.

Arterial pulsations can be graded on the basis of 0 to 4. Grade 0 signifies a complete absence of pulsations, indicating the possibility of marked arteriosclerosis; grade 1, a barely palpable pulsation, indicating marked impairment; grade 2, slightly more palpable pulsation, indicating moderate impairment; grade 3, fairly good quality pulsations, indicating slightly impaired blood flow; and grade 4, good quality pulsations, indicating normal blood flow.[7] I would like to point out once again that the presence of hair does not rule out the presence of vascular insufficiency. Elsewhere in the text I will show gangrenous lesions and hair growth co-existing in the same foot.

Edema

The prudent podiatrist always observes the foot of the diabetic for the presence of edema. It is important to realize that arterial impairment does not result in unilateral or bilateral edema of the feet. Some of the common causes for bilateral edema in the diabetic are renal impairment, congestive heart failure (uncompensated), severe malnutrition, and chronic venous insufficiency. Unilateral edema may be caused by thrombophlebitis or phlebothrombosis. In the male with unilateral edema, one must be aware that neoplastic disease of the prostate must be ruled out. Edema caused by chronic venous insufficiency will be a brawny type of edema, frequently accompanied by pigmentation of the skin of the leg. It is felt that this pigmentation is due to the deposition of hemosiderin in the epidermis. Table 1-1 is a guide to the understanding of the broad picture of edema.

TESTS THAT REQUIRE SPECIAL INSTRUMENTS

The Oscillometer

The oscillometer is a very useful instrument in determining the adequacy of the peripheral blood flow. I should like to point out that the oscillometer can be misused. It can be applied with poor technique and an erroneous result will be observed. The cuff must be applied as tightly as possible before inflation. It is important to remember that the oscillometer should be used at three levels when examining the diabetic foot. One must take oscillometric readings below both knees, above each ankle, and in both feet. One then compares the various excursions of the oscillometer at various levels. I would like to point out that a reading of 6 below the right knee and a reading of 2 at the right ankle would be normal if one did not take the left side and find the left side to be 10 below the

Table 1-1. A Guide to the Etiology of Edema

1. Increase in venous pressure
   a. Congestive heart failure
   b. obstruction to venous flow (phlebitis)
   c. neoplasm compressing venous flow
   d. pregnancy
   e. scar tissue within the venous wall
   f. pericarditis
   g. varices
   h. arterio-venous aneuryism
2. Increase in permeability of capillary wall
   a. nephritis
   b. infection
   c. anoxemia
   d. liberation of histamine
   e. vasculitis
3. Decrease in osmotic pressure
   a. hypoproteinemia
   b. loss of blood
   c. protein starvation
   d. diarrhea
   e. cirrhosis of the liver
4. Increase in arteriolar hydrostatic pressure
   a. dilatation of the artioles
   b. avitaminosis (beri-beri)
5. Lymphedema
   a. inflammatory
   b. non-inflammatory

knee and 4 at the ankle. Thus, it is evident that one must take bilateral readings and compare the bilateral readings to ascertain vascular deficiencies in one limb.

The Doppler Apparatus

Using the Doppler flow meter, the podiatrist can actually hear the blood flow in the peripheral vessels. A gel is liberally applied over the dorsum of the foot. The earphones are placed on the head of the examiner at the same time that he gently places the diaphragm on the foot covered with the gel. The examiner listens very carefully for the "swish," or actual sound, of the coursing blood in the dorsalis pedis artery. Gel is now placed posterior to the medial malleolus and again the Doppler diaphragm head is gently moved in the area of the normal pathway of the posterior tibial artery. The trained observer will be able to differentiate the arterial sound from the venous sound. The venous sound is much softer. The same procedure can be carried out in the popliteal space and in the inguinal triangle.

The clinician, by placing three pneumatic cuffs on the lower extremity, can determine the level of obstruction. Basically, the procedure is carried out by first inflating the pneumatic cuff above the systolic level just above the ankle. He slowly deflates the cuff and listens for the return or absence of the dorsalis pedis and posterior tibial arteries. The same procedure is repeated sequentially below the knee and above the knee. It is important to repeat the procedure at the same three levels in both extremities. One can confirm one's physical findings with any conventional oscillometer, and in fact, they should be used jointly.

The Arteriogram

When frank gangrene or severe ischemic rest pain is present in a limb, it is incumbent upon the attending physician and the attending podiatrist to ask for and receive arteriograms of both limbs. This technique is carried out by the radiologist. A radio-opaque dye is injected into the femoral artery and the vascular tree is visualized. One can see the level of obstruction. The clinician can also determine the absence or presence of a good "run-off". This will indicate to the vascular surgeon whether arterial reconstruction is in order or whether, in fact, arterial reconstruction would be a useless procedure. The arteriogram is not, however, foolproof. Like any modality, it is but one factor to be added to the physical work-up prior to clinical judgment.

The X-ray

Radiography, as we know, is a very useful modality in the management of the diabetic foot. It must be pointed out, however, that a radiogram can be misleading. Early in the clinical picture of osteomyelitis, X-rays of the osseous structures may be entirely free of the condition. Competent radiologists may interpret osteomyelitis as "negative for bony pathology". I emphasize that

18

early in the disease there is no lytic process that can be seen on X-ray. It is always safe to asssume that if a sinus tract has osseous tissue as its base, we are dealing with osteomyelitis. In other words, if you can pass a sterile probe into a sinus tract and palpate bone, that bone is infected. A negative X-ray does not mean that we are not dealing with bony pathology.

Early detection of Charcot foot is extremely difficult by the use of X-ray. We all are familiar with the "bag of bones" that is clearly Charcot's foot in the neuropathic diabetic foot. I have constantly found that the proximal phalanges of the neuropathic foot give a most important clue. Early in the disease, prior to the obvious massive osseous changes which we refer to as Charcot's foot, the proximal phalanges of the lesser toes show an "hourglass" type of deformity. The diaphysis becomes narrow, making the phalanx appear hour-glassed.

The X-ray can pick up marked, uniform calcification of the media of large and small arteries. This calcification, which is within the arterial wall, is commonly referred to as Monckeberg's arteriosclerosis. The lumen is not narrowed or encroached upon. The artery does, however, lose some of its elasticity. In times of stress or exercise, when an increase in blood volume is needed, it is not forthcoming. At this point, the patient may have signs of claudication. The X-ray per se cannot pick up atheramatous plaques which appear on the intima and encroach upon the lumen of the artery.

Vibrometry

The tuning fork must be a part of the podiatrist's equipment if he is treating the diabetic foot. The proper application of the tuning fork can rule in or rule out the presence of peripheral neuropathy. The diabetic foot is likely to be affected.

Culture and Sensitivity Studies

When the diabetic presents himself for treatment of a lesion, it is necessary for the podiatrist to take a sample of the exudate and attempt to culture the microorganism. When the organism has been cultured, it may be identified and exposed to a battery of antibiotics. In this manner we can establish, in vitro, the explicit antibiotic to vigorously treat the patient. It is wise, from a medical-legal point of view, to have a licensed medical laboratory determine the specific microorganism and the effective antibiotic. Culture and sensitivity studies should be repeated if the clinical picture does not improve. I have found that the organism may become resistant to one particular antibiotic after several days of oral or parenteral therapy.

The podiatrist should order culture and sensitivity studies of anaerobic as well as aerobic bacteria. All suspicious nails should be cultured for mycotic disease. Often the potassium hydroxide preparation does not show mycelia, but Sabouraud's agar or an enriched media reveal a mycotic infection.

REFERENCES

1. Conrad, M.C.: *Functional Anatomy of the Circulation to the Lower Extremities*, Year Book Medical Publishers, Chicago, 1971.

2. Grant, J.C.B., and Couper, J.: *The Anatomy of Blood Vessels and Lymphatic Systems*, Oxford University Press, New York, 1957.

3. Geiringer, E.: Intimal vascularization and atherosclerosis. *Journal of Pathology and Bacteriology*, **63**:201–211, 1951.

4. Lewis, T.: Observation on reactions of blood vessels. *Heart*, **15**:177–208, 1930.

5. Collens, W.S., and Wilensky, D.: *Peripheral Vascular Disease*, 2nd Edition, Charles C. Thomas, Springfield, Illinois, 1953.

6. Rakow, R.B., and Friedman, S.A.: The significances of graphic foot changes in the aged. *Geriatrics*, **24**:135, 1969.

7. Allen, E.V., Barker, N.W., and Hines, E.A.: *Peripheral Vascular Diseases*, Third Edition, W.B. Saunders, Philadelphia, 1962.

CHAPTER 2

Care of the Diabetic Foot

THE FOOT WITH NO APPARENT LESIONS

From the outset one should realize that there is no such thing as routine care of the diabetic foot. The diabetic foot must be treated with maximum tenderness, and the minimum of trauma. One must be aware of the fact that the palpating finger on a distal end of a digit (or on any part of the foot) that is vascularly impaired can cause necrosis.

All instruments to be used in caring for the patient must be sterilized and individually packed. Cold sterilization with any of the commercial products on the market is adequate for this purpose. All the toes should be thoroughly and carefully washed with a detergent. Follow this with a liberal amount of alcohol applied to the toes, to the clavi, and to the tyloma. The nails, as they need care, should be cut with a sterile nail cutter, leaving no denuded areas. One should not be heroic in removing nail spicules, nor should one traumatize the nail fold of the diabetic foot. When treating tylomata and clavi one must realize that all the hyperkerotic tissues should not be removed. It is wise to leave a safe level or a base of the original callus tissue in site. After the nails, the tylomata and the clavi have been reduced, a suitable antiseptic is applied. If possible, any adhesive dressing should be avoided when dealing with the diabetic foot. It is not necessary to don sterile gloves prior to the reduction of the excrescence. It is most important, however, to have the operator scrub his hands for five minutes in the same fashion he would for any type of surgery.

Onychogryphotic nails may be the media for mycotic invasion. Using an electrically driven burr, only the excess nail plate is

21

removed. Extreme caution must be exercised when using the motor driven burr. The diabetic foot is all too often impaired vis-a-vis heat sensation. It is possible to cause thermal necrosis without the patient feeling the "burn".

I emphasize again that there are no routine diabetic feet. There is no routine care given to the diabetic foot. Every diabetic foot needs special care, special instrumentation, and close observation. One must remember that if a nail is cut too deeply by the patient, by the patient's family, or even professionally, the result can be an infection. The infection can result in a gangrenous lesion. The gangrenous lesion can result in an amputation.

The podiatrist is taught to use the scalpel, or the instrument he may prefer, in reducing excrescences. Nothing is ever mentioned with regard to the other hand of the operator, the one not holding the instrument. The skilled podiatrist makes certain that he never grasps, or in any way causes trauma to, the patient's foot. A good guide is the following: If you are holding the patient's foot with enough tension or pressure to cause blanching in the nail beds of your fingers, you are placing entirely too much pressure on the patient's foot. This pressure is enough to cause local necrosis.

The podiatrist attempting to care for the diabetic patient must be aware of the risk he assumes. The diabetic patient must be informed that he is, indeed, in a class by himself. Podiatry's major contribution to the health care of the community is to prevent, if possible, and therefore lower the rate of amputations.

THE FOOT WITH ARTERIOSCLEROSIS OBLITERANS

It is abundantly clear that the principal reason for amputation is arterial insufficiency. I agree with Ecker and Jacobs[1] that the accepted philosophy has been to try to make the first amputation the patient's only amputation. Unfortunately, this is not the case. Despite marked improvement in surgical skill, atherosclerosis is still responsible for failures and revision of surgical procedures. When the cure for, or the method for prevention of, gangrene is discovered, it will be in the prevention of atherosclerosis and/or the reversibility of the occlusion or narrowing of the blood vessel. I feel this is a metabolic process, perhaps under the influence of the endocrine system, in an organ or organs not indicted as yet. The cure is not in the surgical correction of the defects that have already made their mark on all of the arterial tree.

One hundred and fifteen years ago, Marchal de Calvi noted that surgery for gangrene of one leg does not alter the prognosis for gangrene in the opposite member.[2] In 1959, Goldner[3] called to our attention the fact that the presence of a gangrenous lesion in one foot or leg precedes the development of gangrene in the contralateral limb. In the Goldner series, 50 percent of his patients developed gangrene in the other limb within two years after involvement of the first limb. Only three patients, after five years, did not have frank gangrene in the remaining limb. It is interesting to note that the remaining three had reduced oscillometric readings in the remaining limb. Foreboding, to say the least. Ecker and Jacobs reported in 1970[1], in their series of 43 bilateral amputees, that the second amputation occurred within two years of the first amputation in twenty-six patients. In summary, over 60% of patients having one leg removed can expect to lose the remaining limb within two years of the first surgical amputation.

One can answer in the affirmative if asked, "With reasonable medical certainty, can you say the patient will develop gangrene in his other leg?" In my experience, which encompasses 35 years of active hospital practice, I can say without equivocation that frequent regular podiatric care can reduce the rate of amputation. In two large metropolitan hospitals with a patient census of over 15,000 diabetics, we have an amputation rate of less than two percent. This does not mean that the diabetic population does not develop ulcerations and gangrene of the toes. It does mean that with regular, frequent podiatric care, the rate of amputations does not have to be in the order of 50 percent. It can be, and is, markedly reduced. The key, other than excellent care, is regular frequent podiatric care. It is time that physicians and the laity realize that there is a profession entirely devoted to the care of an organ of the body, the foot.

THE FOOT WITH MECHANICAL DEFECTS

The care of mechanical defects which commonly occur in the diabetic foot is a serious problem. The podiatrist must be certain that the orthotic, appliance or device is not causing pressure on any area of the foot. As a general rule, I would advocate the use of such material as plastozote, rubber butter or leather. If the problem is basically one of rearfoot or forefoot malposition, the podiatrist may choose to employ posted orthotics. He must, however, make certain that the shoes accommodate the orthotic and that no pressure is exerted on either the rearfoot or the forefoot. A word of caution: If you elect to use a plastozote mould appliance, do not heat the plastozote and have the patient step onto the material. It is possible to cause thermal necrosis with this technique. Remember, the diabetic patient is not aware of possible harmful temperature ranges due to an overt or covert neuropathy. It is always wise to first take a negative plaster of Paris cast. Convert the negative cast to a positive one. Using the positive impression of the patient's foot, press the cast unto the plastozote, thereby creating the same orthotic without the hazard of burning the patient.

Under the heading of general care of the diabetic foot, I think it proper to discuss the moulded shoe. A great many of our patients have inoperable deformities of the feet. The concept of a custom made shoe is a good one. The end product may be a catastrophe. The shoes fit the patient like a glove. The marked hallux valgus deformity is accommodated. The dorsally dislocated toes remain dislocated. The glaring fault is that the shoe should not fit like a glove. The foot at the end of the day is larger than at the beginning of the working day. The foot has become edematous. I am not referring to the obvious pitting edema. I mean the minute, subtle edema that the patient will develop during the day. The shoe, however, does not become larger. Pressure necrosis and gangrene of the dorsal and distal aspect of the toes can occur.

REFERENCES

1. Ecker, M.L., and Jacobs, B.S.: Lower extremity amputation in diabetic patients. *Diabetes,* **19**:189, 1970.
2. Marchal de Calvi, C.J.: *Recherches sur les Accidents Diabetiques,* P. Asselin, Paris, 1864.
3. Goldner, M.G.: The fate of the second leg in the diabetic amputee. *Diabetes,* **9**:100, 1960.

CHAPTER 3

Avoiding Malpractice Suits

Any podiatrist who has had experience in this field will know full well the importance of a proper history. First, I would like to re-emphasize that there is no "routine" podiatric care for the diabetic patient. If the patient is in your office for treatment of an excrescence or a functional deformity, you must record a legible history and physical examination. When the patient with frank gangrene or ulceration requests podiatric treatment, the picture is entirely changed.

Second, the patient with lesions may lose a toe, a foot, a limb or his life. This patient cannot be treated as an ambulatory patient. This risk is far too great. He must be hospitalized. Therefore, every podiatrist who treats the diabetic must have co-admitting privileges to a hospital.

When the patient is admitted to the hospital, have a written consultation with a board certified internist. This consultation will reflect the general condition and the diabetic status of the patient. It is also important to have a written consultation with a specialist in vascular diseases.

It is important and imperative that the podiatrist do a culture and sensitivity study on all patients with open lesions. Oscillometric readings, venous filling time and, in fact, a complete vascular work-up should be done on all diabetic patients with lesions.

Thirdly, if a patient should refuse hospitalization, he must sign a written document which will point out that the podiatrist has ordered the patient to the hospital and the patient in fact refuses to go.

It is wise to X-ray both feet of the patient with a lesion. Often one detects the presence of Charcot foot, osteoporosis, calcified vessels, neoplastic disease (osseogenic sarcoma or osteomyelitis) or fractures when X-raying both feet. When the patient has been hospitalized, it may be wise to order arteriograms. The ordering of arteriograms may not be within the domain of the podiatrist. The podiatrist should be aware of the fact that the co-admitting physician should order the arteriograms, because he is just as liable for malpractice as the podiatrist if he does not. If arteriography is not done, the reason for failure to carry it out should be noted on the hospital chart. One of the reasons for failure to do an arteriogram is that the patient refuses. One may not order an arteriogram if the patient is too sick to undergo the rigors of the examination. Whatever the reason may be, it must be noted on the hospital chart. It is wise to take pictures of all lesions from the first day. One must indicate on the patient's chart the exact day the picture was taken and, if possible, have the patient sign a document indicating that a photo was taken on such a date. (I have deliberately repeated myself for the sake of emphasis.)

One must always indicate the size of the lesion, the depth of the lesion, the character of the lesion, and the texture and quality of surrounding skin. It is important to know the age of the lesion and, if possible, the etiology of the lesion.

In dealing with a diabetic patient who has occlusive vascular disease, one must always give a guarded or frankly poor prognosis. One must treat every patient as if he or she were going to lose his/her limb. No one ever cures an easy case of gangrene. The podiatrist must explain to the patient's family that the prognosis is poor, that he is trying all known methods, that he will call in all consultants and make every effort to avert an amputation and a calamity. It is important never to discredit another practitioner. Notes on your chart should never be changed once they are written. An attorney can go over your notes and find that you've changed a three to an eight or a two to a four, and the credibility of the entire document goes down the drain. Make notes on your chart every day. Do not wait until the end of the week to fill in an entire charting progression of symptoms. Be sure that the dates are correct and are in proper sequence. Remember that it is the prerogative of every and any patient to sue the podiatrist, the physician, the hospital, or anyone remotely connected with the case. In this day and age, with malpractice suits constantly on the rise, the podiatrist should be aware of the necessity of a proper history, a proper physical, and proper documentation of every diabetic case with a lesion that he treats. If the podiatrist has proper and thorough documentation of every incident at the hospital and every change in the clinical picture, he is protected.

The following can serve as a guide. It is intended for all podiatrists treating the diabetic lesion.

• Hospitalize the patient.

• Complete proper physical and work-up, including complete blood count, sequential multiple analysis (SMA 12), electrocardiogram, chest plate.

• Have proper consultation.

• Take fractional urine.

• Do culture and sensitivity studies.

• Order complete bed rest for the patient.

• Order appropriate antibiotic therapy in clinical doses sufficient to affect the clinical picture of the patient. If the patient is on nephrotoxic drugs, order daily blood urea nitrogen.

• Make proper notes on the chart — this is of paramount importance.

• If alkaline phosphatase is elevated, differentiate liver from bone diseases by heating specimen — bone is heat labile, liver is heat stabile.

• Take pictures of the lesion on the first day, and every four to five days thereafter.

A serial study of the patient's progress can be noted in this way and become part of the patient's record. In the event that the patient goes downhill, and does lose his limb, the podiatrist protects himself by documenting the daily progress of the patient. He will then have not only his verbal impression of the clinical picture, he will actually have a photo of the lesion.

A word concerning consultation is in order at this time. The podiatrist should seek out only those physicians who are accredited in their particular specialty. Every good hospital has just such a list of medical specialists. The consultation and his recommendations become part and parcel of the patient's record.

In the event that the patient fails to follow the orders of the podiatrist or the physician during his hospital stay, this, likewise, should be documented in the chart. Many times the patient refuses to stay in bed and does ambulate. This violation of orders must become part of the hospital record. There is the occasion when the patient refuses to take his medication. This, likewise, should be documented in the patient's chart. A well-meaning relative often brings in "goodies" for the patient who is hospitalized. This is in violation of good care of the patient. This, too, should be documented in the patient's chart. The patient's family is violating hospital laws and your orders by bringing in food. This clearly points out the patient's lack of cooperation and indicts the patient's family if a failure should occur.

CHAPTER 4

Cutaneous Disorders of the Diabetic Foot

Before discussing the common skin disorders to which the diabetic is heir, it is necessary to review the micro-anatomy and the physiology of the skin.

The skin is an organ of the body with specific functions that we are all aware of. For our purposes, it is very important to remember that the skin is a storage reservoir for glucose. Only the liver can store a greater amount of glucose. It is, therefore, evident that the skin is an adjunct organ in maintaining glucose levels. Fusaro and Johnson[1] have shown that after the intravenous injection of glucose, 15% of the blood glucose can be detected in the dermis. The maximum glucose level in the dermis is reached in one-half hour. The normal blood sugar returns to its prefasting level in one hour. It is most important to note, however, that the glucose level in the dermis does not return to its prefasting level for two to three hours. In other words, the dermis can be a slow, constant source of glucose to the blood.

It is important to know that glucose leaves the dermis at a much slower rate in the diabetic patient as compared to the non-diabetic. Fusaro[2] states that glucose disappears from the dermis at the rate of 0.3% per minute. The normal patient shows a dermal glucose loss rate of 2% per minute.[3] One can, in the light of this knowledge, readily see that the dermis in the diabetic patient becomes a very fine culture medium for pathogenic microorganisms. Bacteria and Candida prefer glucose as their source of energy. It is now clear why we see so many infections of the foot and, further, why the incidence of foot infections in the diabetic is as large as we know it to be.

The diabetic foot is indeed prone to bacterial infection, mycotic infection and Candida. Bacterial infection is commonly seen in the nail groove. When it occurs at this site, paronychia is the diagnosis most often given. The etiology is most often self-induced trauma when the patient attempts to cut his nail. I have seen many "well meant" iatrogenically-induced paronychia subsequent to "professional" treatment of an ingrowing toe nail. Ingrowing toe nail and paronychia are not to be taken lightly when they occur in the diabetic. The skin should be sterilized with ethyl alcohol and sterile nail cutter and nail chisel are used to remove only the spicule of nail that has become caught in the nail flap. Under no circumstances should the toe be blocked with a local anesthetic. If the podiatrist is causing sufficient pain to call for a local anesthetic, he is not performing with the best of podiatric skills. Following the removal of the spicule of nail, it is wise to do culture and sensitivity studies with the purulent exudate. Before the laboratory reports the proper antibiotic, I suggest you prescribe a broad spectrum antibiotic (see section on antibiotics). I have recently seen a patient who had the nail bed removed on the first visit for paronychia. The podiatrist was told the patient had diabetes. This course of management is indefensible. It is not accepted podiatric procedure to remove the nail bed of a diabetic as a means to cure a paronychia. It is not uncommon to find ingrowing toe nails and paronychia on any and all of the lesser toes.

Onychomycosis is perhaps the second most common infection involving the nail plate. Here we usually find more than one toe affected. The nail is thick, discolored and has a characteristic musty odor. Scrapings of the nail plate inoculated on Sabouraud's media will identify the fungus. KOH slide preparation will show the characteristic hyphae (see Figures 1 and 2). The fungi most often identified with mycotic infections are Trichophyton rubrum and Trichophyton mentagrophytes.

One must keep in mind that darkness, heat and moisture make for an ideal setting for the fungi to make inroads. The interdigital spaces are prime sites for mycotic infections. While griseofulvin by mouth and topical clotrimazole (Lotrimin®) are effective in the management of mycotic infections in the diabetic, I have found preventive measures to be very efficient. First and foremost, the patient should have a daily foot bath. This may sound trite and repetitious. "Vagabond's disease," or lack of bathing, is just as common in the diabetic population as in the general population. The feet should be thoroughly dried by gently patting the interspaces and not by pulling a thick towel between the toes. Socks in the summer should be of cotton only. In the winter, only wool stockings are to be worn. No synthetic material should be considered by the diabetic when he or she purchases stockings. Shoes should, preferably, be made of soft kid skin. Man-made leather shoes should not be worn by the diabetic. One cannot recommend any brand of shoe. The prime consideration in the purchase of shoes should be left to the discretion of a skilled, honest, conscientious shoe fitter. This individual is most rare today.

Candida infections are commonly seen in the interdigital areas of the feet. The podiatrist may be the first health professional to detect diabetes if he recognizes a Candida infection. The skin is usually white, moist and exfoliating. Pruritis may or may not be present. It is wise to ask the patient if he or she has a similar dermatitis elsewhere. The groin, the axilla and beneath pendulous breasts are frequent sites for Candida infections. Treatment is usually nystatin. I have been successful using topical clotrimazole (Lotrimin®) solution.

The podiatrist should be aware of the fact that any infection of the foot can cause the diabetes to become out of control. While it is altogether fitting and proper for the podiatrist to treat the local foot infection, he should alert the patient and the patient's physician. The glycosuria and the glycemia must be carefully monitored during this time.

Other skin lesions seen on the foot and leg of the diabetic patient include dermopathy[4] or brown spots. These occur on the anterior of the leg and serve only to give the patient cause for needless concern. It can be theorized that these are caused by the leakage of hemosiderin into the subcutaneous tissue by capillaries that have become brittle. It is wise to instruct the patient to protect the area from trauma and avoid exposure to the sun.

The most frequent epidermal pathology encountered on the diabetic foot is the callus. The thickening of the stratum corneum can be seen at any location on the foot. It is most frequently seen at the heads of the metatarsal bones; however, it can occur at any site. Common areas are over bony prominences. A contributing factor in their formation is the atrophy of the natural adipose tissue usually located on the plantar aspect of the foot.

It is usual and customary to reduce the excess keratotic tissue under aseptic technique with a minimum of trauma. It is best to

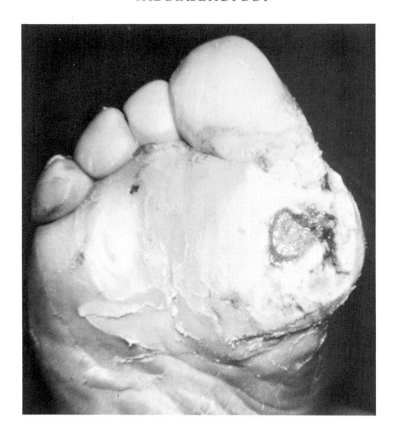

Figure 3. Diabetic ulcer caused by pressure and salicylic acid.

employ a sterile scalpel for this purpose. The area under reduction should be liberally sprayed with alcohol or another suitable antiseptic while the podiatrist is working. It is not wise to cover the site of the callus with moleskin or other adhesive. It is not uncommon to find maceration and areas of allergic response when an adhesive dressing is used following reduction of a hyperkeratotic area.

The use of a pumice stone is to be condemned. I have seen gangrene develop in areas previously attacked with an abrasive stone. The use of salicylic acid pads are to be condemned. The use of preparations containing salicylic acid cause chemical burns. The patient in Figures 3, 4 and 5 is a fifty-nine year old female. She was known to have diabetes mellitus for fifteen years. She was main-

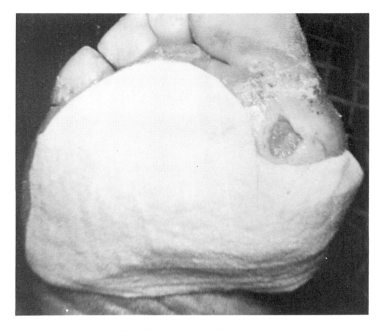

Figure 4. Shielding with felt to allow ambulation.

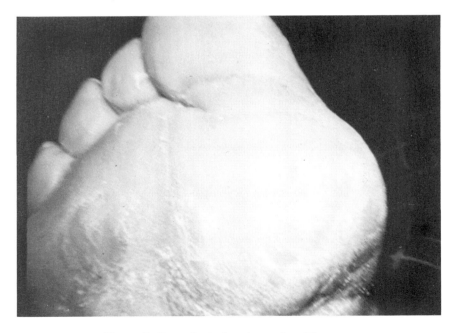

Figure 5. Same foot after six weeks of therapy.

tained on daily injections of NPH insulin. The internist adjusted her dose, which ranged from 20 units to 40 units. She was complaining of callus formation for "years". In an attempt to reduce her medical bills, she applied a commercial product designed to rid her of her callus. The result was an infected callus ulcer with an area of necrosis. Adequate antibiotic therapy, removal of weight bearing and appropriate debridement resulted in a cure of the gangrene and infection. Proper orthotic therapy did not relieve her of the callus problem. It did, however, allow her to function normally, and ten years after this episode she has not had a recurrence of the ulceration.

The formation of clavi or "corns" on the dorsal aspect of the toes can be a source of infection and gangrene in the diabetic foot. Neither the patient nor his family should ever attempt to remove the excrescence by any means. A common sequence of events following the use of corn plasters or an abrasive board is shown in Figures 6 through 11. The patient in these figures is a sixty year old diabetic female. Her vascular supply was within normal limits. Her diabetes was controlled by the use of insulin mixtures (regular 10 units, protamine 20 units) injected daily before breakfast. An ulceration developed on the dorsal aspect of the right fourth toe following the use of a commercial product containing salicylic acid in solution. As you will note in Figure 7, the ulcerated area has developed a sinus tract which emerged on the lateral aspect of the toe. Figures 8 and 9 demonstrate the use of a drain (through and through) to effect adequate drainage. (Appropriate therapy will be discussed in Chapters 9 and 10.) Figures 10 and 11 were taken eight weeks after the onset of therapy.

Necrobiosis lipoidica also occurs on the anterior surface of the legs. These superficial lesions are usually 1 cm to 3 cm in diameter. The skin is atrophic and pigmented. The lesions may appear as a single patch, or they may be multiple in character. These are benign and are of no significance other than being cosmetically objectionable. I have excised a benign xanthoma from the plantar aspect of the foot of a twenty-nine year old female diabetic.

Verruca plantaris are quite rare in the diabetic. I feel this may be due to the quality of foot hygiene usually given to the diabetic foot. In patients with normal vascularity, the treatment can be either electrical or chemical cautery. In patients with impaired

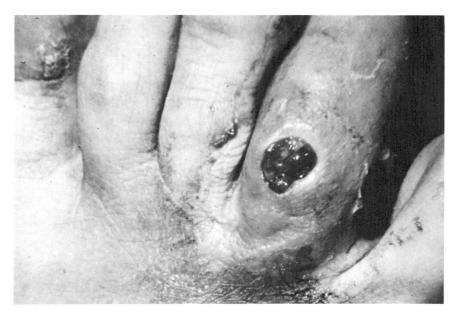

Figure 6. Ulcer on dorsal aspect of right fourth toe penetrating to bone, causing an exogenous osteomyelitis.

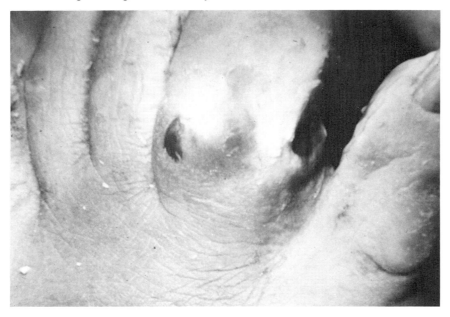

Figure 7. Lesion moved from dorsum to lateral aspect of toes.

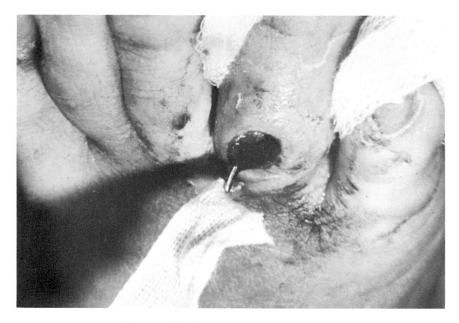

Figure 8. A through and through drain.

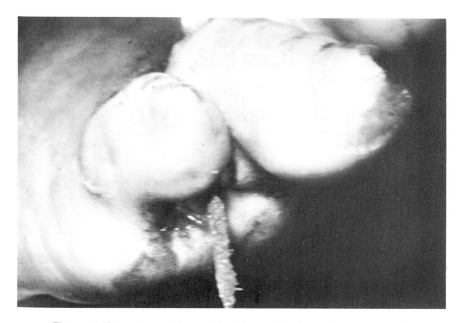

Figure 9. Through and through iodoform drain from dorsum, emerging from lateral aspect of the fourth toe.

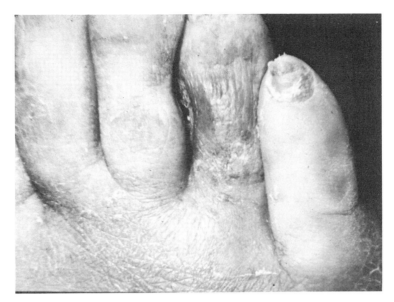

Figure 10. Lesion healed, normal function, patient working without loss of digit.

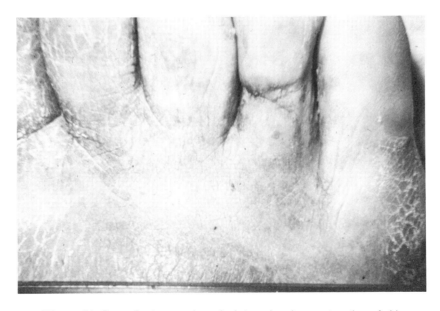

Figure 11. Same foot several weeks later, showing contraction of skin.

vascularity, one should remove weight bearing by means of an orthotic.

Heel fissures, while appearing to be benign, are the source of many gangrenous heels.

REFERENCES

1. Fusaro, R.M., and Johnson, J.A.: The dermal glucose compartment. In Montagna, E.W. (Ed.): *Advances in Biology of Skin*, Vol. 10, New York, Appleton-Century-Crofts (in press).
2. Fusaro, R.M.: *Some Aspects of Glucose Kinetics and Metabolism in the Skin*. Doctoral thesis, University of Minnesota Medical School, Minneapolis, 1965.
3. Fusaro, R.M.[1] and Goetz, F.C.: *Common Cutaneous Manifestations and Problems of Diabetes Mellitus*. Doctoral thesis, University of Minnesota Medical School, Minneapolis, 1965.
4. Melin, H: An atrophic circumscribed skin lesion in the lower extremities of diabetics. *Acta Med. Scand.*, **176**:Suppl 423: 1, 1964.

CHAPTER 5

Neurological Findings In The Diabetic Foot

The term *diabetic osteopathy* has been used to describe a variety of poorly understood destructive bone changes seen in the feet of patients with diabetes mellitus. Since these lesions are generally associated with significant peripheral neuropathy, it seems reasonable to assume that the two are etiologically related, but the precise relationship is still unclear. The demonstration of similar bone findings in leprosy[1] suggests that osteopathy is a result of neurological impairment rather than a co-existing effect of a metabolic disturbance of diabetes mellitus. It is possible that the loss of pain and proprioceptive sensation makes the bone prone to trauma because of insidious changes in stance and gait that may cause prolonged and excessive pressure on certain parts of the foot.[2] On the other hand, it has been suggested that autosympathectomy secondary to neuropathy may lead to small vessel dilation and encourage the resorption of bone.[3]

DIABETIC OSTEOPATHY

Neurotrophic skeletal change in the feet of patients with diabetes mellitus is a recognized clinical entity,[3-8] but much confusion exists concerning its frequency, etiology and significance. In seeing patients with diabetic peripheral neuropathy, I have been impressed with the extent and frequency of silent bone destruction, especially in the phalanges and metatarsals. These lesions simulate the changes associated with osteomyelitis and may present a clinical dilemma in patients with concomitant epithelial necrosis.

The neurological findings are bilateral and symmetrical in most patients. Positive neurological signs are usually a loss of pain (anesthesia, hypesthesia), loss of light touch, loss of proprioceptive sense and loss of, or diminished, vibratory sense. Knee jerks and ankle jerks are absent or diminished. The patient's feet appear quite warm, with no cutaneous signs of ischemia. Anhydrosis and atrophy of the intrinsic muscles of the feet are not uncommon. Pedal pulses are usually palpable. Oscillometric readings and venous filling time are within normal range.

Radiographic abnormalities tend to have certain distinct patterns in different areas of the foot. In the toes, osteopathy can be evaluated accurately in the proximal phalanges. The phalangeal changes, for the most part, consist of rather symmetrical thinning of the bone, most marked in the center of the metaphysis, with progressively less involvement toward the epiphyses — this change tending to give the appearance of an hourglass. Osteoblastic reaction along the periosteum of the metaphyses is frequent.

In the metatarsal bone, destructive lesions are non-specific. The heads of these bones are most involved, usually with irregular destruction, and occasionally with small punctate areas of bone resorption. The tarsal bones are involved infrequently, the most common site being the cuneiforms and the navicular.

Phalangeal disease is most frequent, but bone destruction is most extensive in the metatarsal bones, an area of the foot that usually absorbs the greatest proportion of the pressure produced in the upright position. On the other hand, the adequacy of the circulation in these patients, in contrast to many other diabetics, might favor bone resorption.[9,10] Although joint destruction may result from osteopathy, it is fundamentally a disease of the entire bone, rather than merely of the periarticular surfaces.[11]

Since relatively little has been written about diabetic osteopathy, its incidence and prevalence are unknown. In one survey of 242 outpatient diabetics, 6.8% had either bone destruction or generalized osteoporosis of the feet.[11] On the other hand, Gondos[12] was able to collect only 36 cases of osteopathy in a review of diabetic patients seen in a large municipal hospital during a ten year period. The present series was accumulated through referral of patients to a peripheral vascular service. It would seem that diabetic osteopathy is a common lesion if 17 cases could be found in this manner in one year, and that it is very frequent in severe diabetic neuropathy. The lesion tends to follow the symmetrical, distal distribution of the neurologic findings, almost always involving the phalanges, usually the metatarsals, and occasionally the tarsal bones.

Although the bone destruction does not produce pain, it may be associated with clinical signs. Club-like deformity of the foot, and signs of an inflammatory response (painless swelling and hyperemia) are frequent occurrences. It is usual to have a normal gait. It is conceivable, however, that deformities produced by bone destruction increase the likelihood of plantar ulceration.

The major clinical significance of diabetic osteopathy is its similarity, in many cases, to osteomyelitis. It is important to distinguish between these two entities in patients with cutaneous lesions, because their prognosis and treatment are quite different. Osteomyelitis in the foot of a diabetic is often associated with impaired arterial circulation, and is difficult to eradicate with antibacterial therapy. When conservative care fails, it may be necessary to resort to surgical attempts to improve the circulation and to exploration of the infected bone and currettage of necrotic fragments. Osteopathy related to denervation does not require any intervention, even if the bone shows progressive changes.

Radiologic distinction is not easy, and often virtually impossible, since resorption and destruction of bone are common to both osteomyelitis and osteopathy. The multifocal involvement, bilaterality and peripheral distribution of the latter are helpful in differential diagnosis. In addition, the symmetrical thinning of the metaphysis, especially in the phalanges, appears to be characteristic of osteopathy. However, the distinction is ultimately a clinical one. A purulent skin ulcer communicating with bone is likely to represent osteomyelitis, even if the X-ray is negative early in the patient's course; but bone changes without this finding should be considered osteopathy until proved otherwise in patients with diabetic neuropathy.

Although diabetic osteopathy is clearly related to peripheral neuropathy, the exact mechanisms can be established only through the study of a large series of diabetic patients. With appropriate clinical and laboratory observations, it can be determined whether osteopathy ever occurs before neuropathy becomes severe, and whether it correlates better with loss of sympathetic or somatic nerve function. The condition appears to be clinically be-

---

Table 5-1. Conditions Compromising the Protective Mechanisms of a Joint

1. Tertiary syphilis
2. Syringomyelia
3. Destructive acropathy, scleroderma, Morvan's disease
4. Peripheral nerve lesions: traumatic, Vitamin B_{12} deficiency
5. Leprosy
6. Poliomyelitis
7. Paraplegia
8. Surgical cordotomy
9. Multiple sclerosis
10. Hereditary sensory radicular neuropathy
11. Intra-articular injection of corticosteroids

---

nign. Long-term prognosis of diabetic osteopathy can be determined only by following patients for many years. Diabetic neuropathy can simulate several other clinical syndromes. Tables 5-1 and 5-2 serve as a guide for differential diagnosis.

CASE HISTORIES OF NEUROPATHY AND LESIONS

Case 1

The patient in Figures 12 through 14 is a fifty year old female physician. She has been a known diabetic for twenty-two years. She has been maintained on N.P.H. insulin daily injection throughout her period of management. X-ray examination (Figure 12) taken on her initial visit shows the characteristic changes of Charcot's disease of the foot. Figure 13 is a photograph taken at the initial visit. She gave a history of self-care for well over one year prior to seeking professional help. Figure 14 is the same foot one month after coming under my care.

She was confined to her house for the entire period of treatment. Treatment included debridement, culture, sensitivity studies and local application of a weak iodine solution. She received oral penicillin (Pen-Vee-K®) one gram per day in divided doses. An appropriate appliance was fitted into her shoe to prevent recurrence. She has not had a recurrence in over one year.

Table 5-2. Conditions Causing Bony Abnormalities Consistent With
or Suggestive of Charcot Joints

1. Acute arthritides
    a. Gout
    b. Acute septic arthritis
    c. Rheumatoid arthritis
2. Chronic pyogenic or tuberculous osteomyelitis
3. Bone tumors
4. Psoriatic arthropathy
5. Vascular insufficiency
6. Osteoarthritis
7. Spina bifida

Case 2

The patient in Figure 15 is a seventy-five year old male with a history of diabetes. Routine X-ray of his right foot shows a foreign body in the foot at the base of the proximal phalanx, in addition to arteriosclerosis of the intermetatarsal arteries. He presented himself for treatment of an ulcer in this area. He denied walking barefooted. The foreign body proved to be a piece of wire.

Basically, we have a diabetic with peripheral arteriosclerosis obliterans. Secondary to this, he has a diabetic neuropathy. He and his family conveniently forget that he walks without shoes and very rarely bathes. If one will observe the third metatarsal bone, one can visualize early neuropathic changes in the head of the metatarsal and similar changes in the base of the proximal phalanx of the third toe. Yet the lesion is at the site of the foreign body, the base of the proximal phalanx of the hallux.

Case 3

The patient in Figures 16 through 18 is a fifty-five year old female. She has had diabetes mellitus for twenty years and has been maintained on insulin therapy throughout the course of her disease.

Figure 16 shows early changes in the toes of the left foot. The second and third toes are dorsally dislocated and the proximal phalanx of the fifth toe is "hourglassed". This is consistent with the diagnosis of Charcot Foot.

43

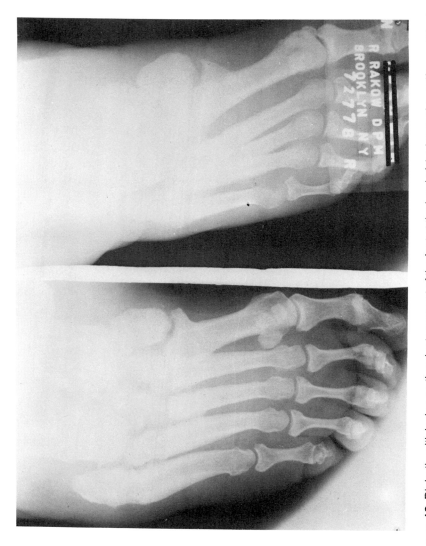

Figure 12. Diabetic with lesion on the plantar aspect of the foot at the level of the internal cuneiform, at the base of the first metatarsal.

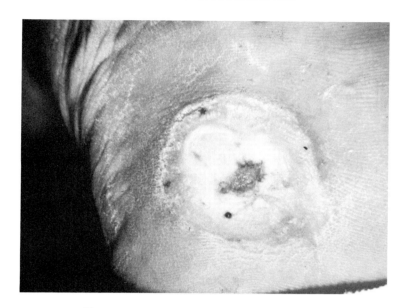

Figure 13. Photograph of lesion in Figure 12.

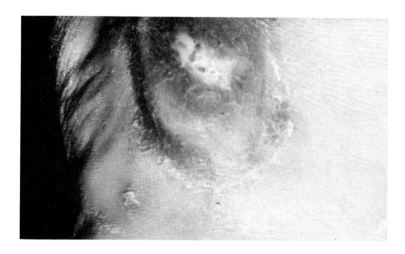

Figure 14. Lesion healed.

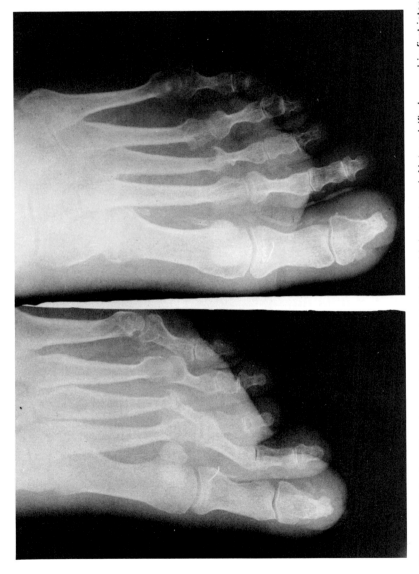

Figure 15. Diabetic with osteomyelitis at the head of the third metatarsal. Note calcified vessel in first inter-metatarsal space. Ulcer due to foreign body at proximal phalanx.

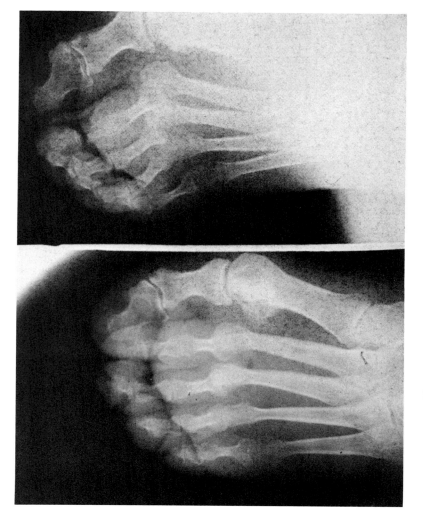

Figure 16. Early changes in foot shown in Figure 15.

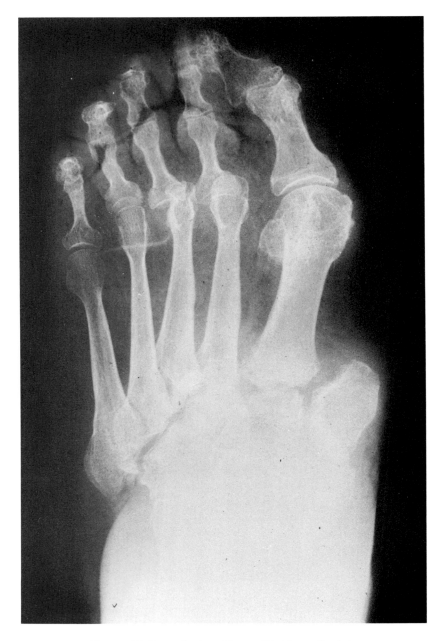

Figure 17. Same foot as Figure 15, 15 months later.

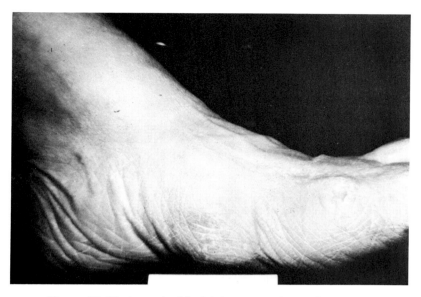

Figure 18. Photograph of foot, taken same day as Figure 17.

Figure 17 is an X-ray of the same foot fifteen months later. We now have the classic bone destruction of Charcot Foot. The tarsometatarsal articulations are affected, in addition to the second and third toes.

Figure 18 is a photograph of the same foot taken the same day as the X-ray in Figure 17. One can clearly see the "rocker" type foot. In effect, the tarsal bones are no longer in their normal alignment. Due to the diabetic neuropathy and resulting alteration in bone metabolism, the massive deformity is now a reality. The patient was totally free of pain. She felt that she had had the usual sequelae to her diabetes mellitus. Other than the unsightly appearance of the foot and the inability to wear stylish shoes, the patient was unimpressed with the X-ray findings.

Case 4

The patient in Figures 19 and 20 is a fifty-two year old male with a history of diabetes mellitus for the past thirty years. He has been maintained on NPH insulin daily since onset of his diabetes. His chief complaint was edema of the great toe of the left foot.

X-ray (Figure 19) revealed the typical Charcot's disease deformity with massive bone destruction. Note the edema of the hallux, the destruction of the base of the distal phalanx, and the destruction of the head, as well as the base, of the proximal phalanx. The third metatarsal head is resorbed and the articulation of the proximal phalanx is destroyed. Also note the hourglass appearance of the proximal phalanges of the fourth and fifth toes.

Figure 20 shows the same patient one year later. There is marked progression of the destruction of the heads of the second and third metatarsal bones. It is interesting to note that this disease is now bilateral. The right foot now shows destruction and resorption of the metatarsal heads.

Case 5

Figure 21 shows Charcot's disease in a sixty year old diabetic. Please observe the toes and metatarsal heads. The patient had no subjective complaints other than painless edema.

Case 6

Figure 22 shows a sixty-five year old female with a twenty-five year history of diabetes, maintained on insulin mixtures. Chief complaint was edema on the dorsum of the right foot with no history of trauma. In addition to the pathological fractures of the second and third metatarsal bones, observe the hourglass deformity of the proximal of the fourth toe.

Case 7

Figure 23 shows a fifty-five year old female with a twenty-five year history of diabetes. She has been maintained on daily injections of protamine insulin since the onset of her diabetes. She reports no subjective symptoms. The figure shows destruction of the second, third and fourth metatarsal bones. The inflammatory reaction in the region of the head of the second metatarsal is typical of the disease. The hourglass or thinning of the metaphyses of the proximal phalanges of the second, third and fourth toes is also seen.

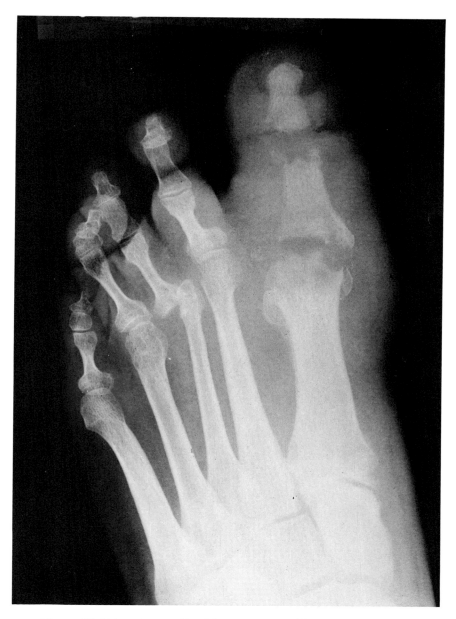

Figure 19. Note osteomyelitis of the great toe and Charcot pathology of the third metatarsal.

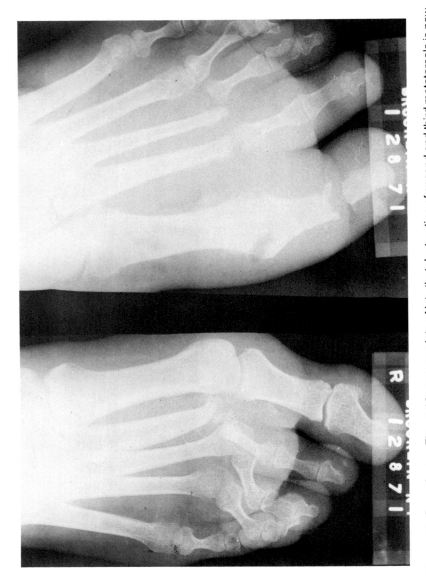

Figure 20. Same foot as Figure 19, one year later. Note that destruction of second and third metatarsals is now bilateral; osteomyelitis is not.

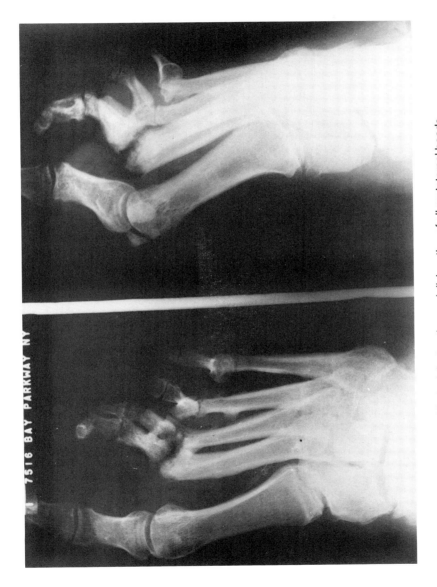

Figure 21. Marked destruction and dislocation of all metatarsal heads.

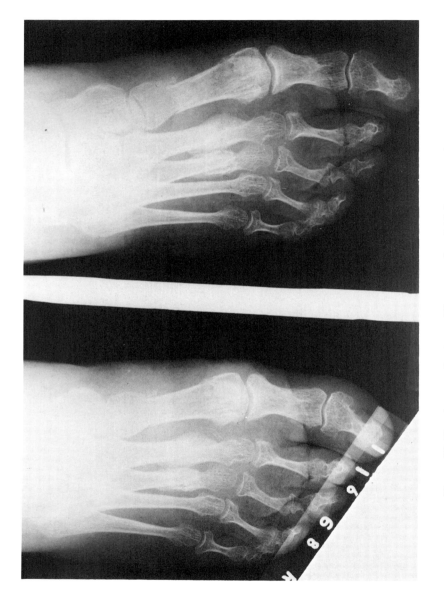

Figure 22. Spontaneous fracture of the second and third metatarsals.

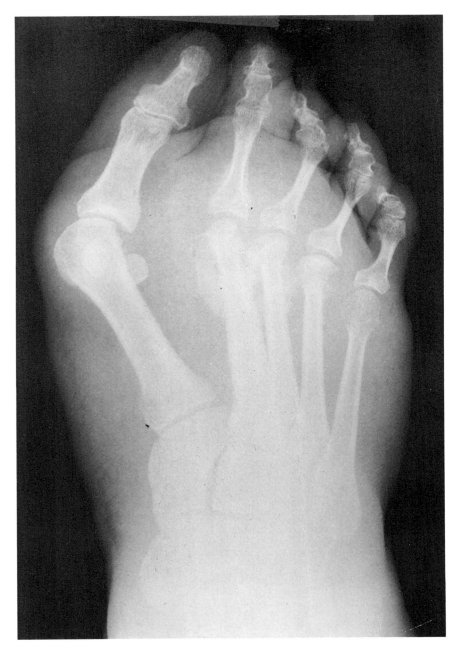

Figure 23. Early Charcot's disease.

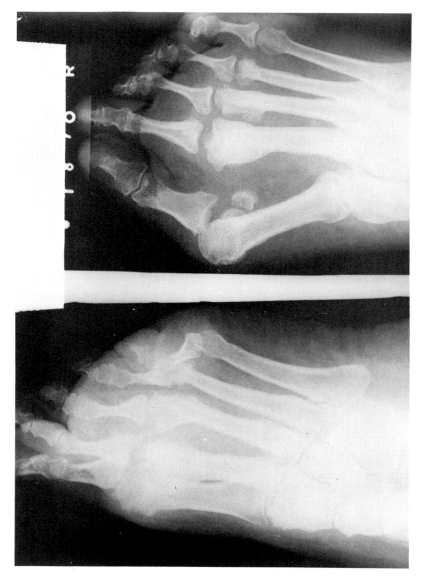

Figure 24. Same foot as in Figure 23, one year later.

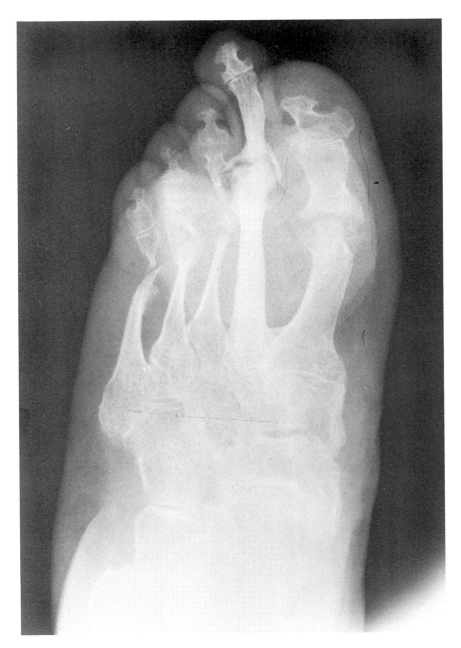

Figure 25. Marked Charcot's disease.

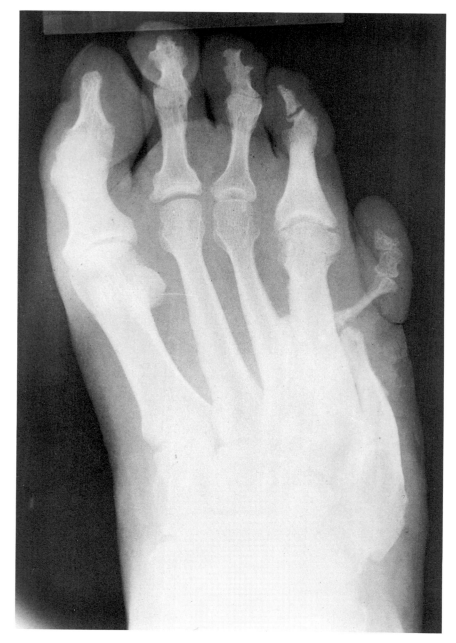

Figure 26. Neurogenic arthropathy in a non-diabetic patient.

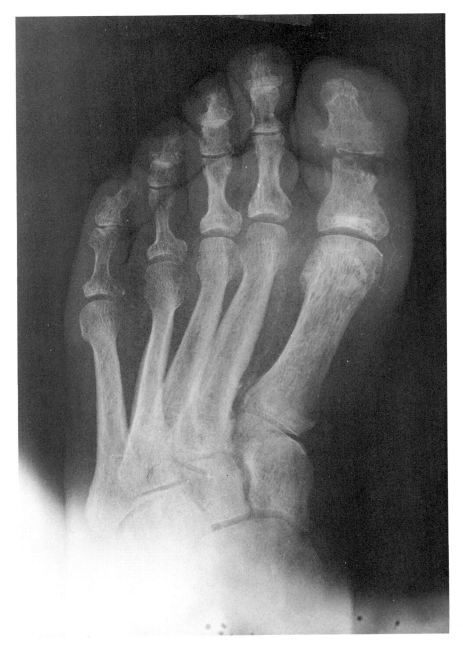

Figure 27. Osteomyelitis: note absence of hourglass effect in phalanges.

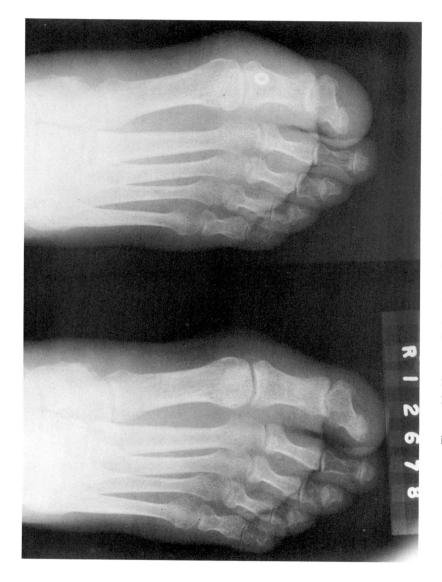

Figure 28. Ulcer on first metatarsal, marked in the photograph.

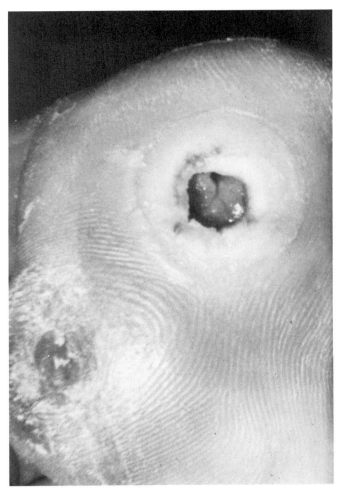

Figure 29. Same patient as Figure 28: deep ulceration eight months later.

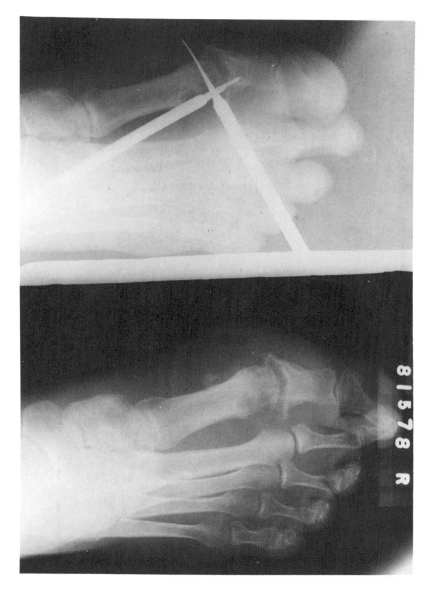

Figure 30: Probes in place at left indicate extent of ulceration. Right X-ray shows marked destruction.

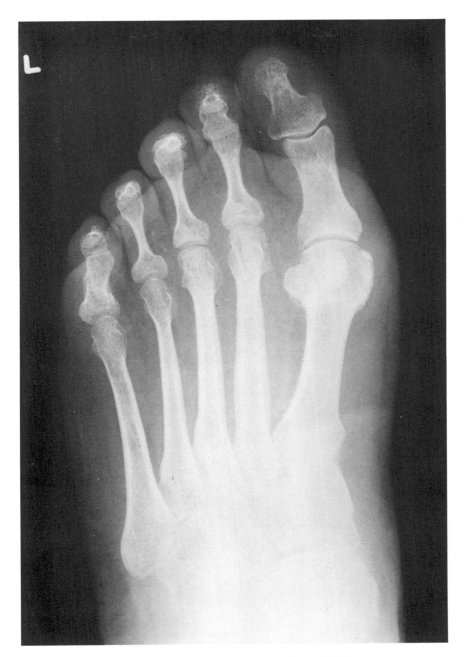

Figure 31. Fracture of proximal phalanx of fifth toe.

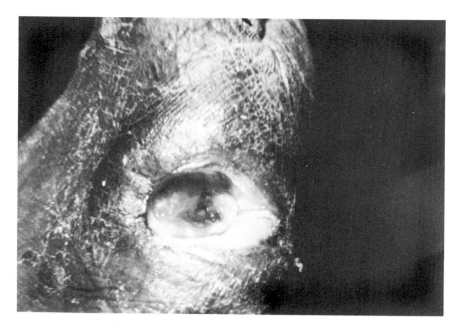

Figure 32. Ulcer at head of fifth metatarsal.

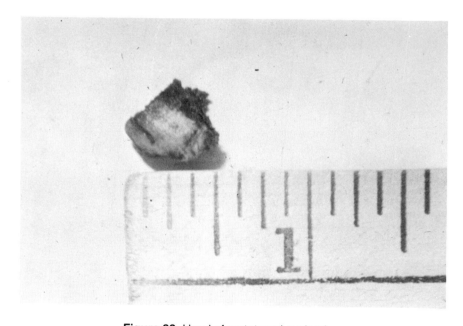

Figure 33. Head of metatarsal excised.

64

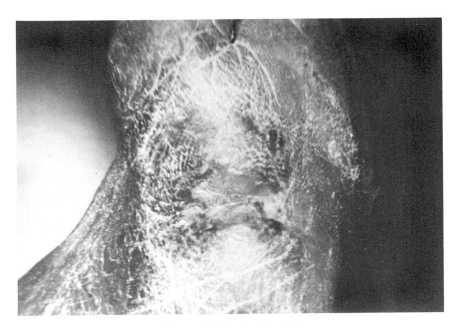

Figure 34. Lesion healed.

Figure 24 shows the same patient one year later. In addition to the progression of the destruction of the metatarsal heads, we can now see the deformity and lateral dislocation of the proximal phalanx of the hallux. At no time did the patient complain of pain. All the neurological findings were positive for Charcot's disease. Her pedal pulses were all present (+4) and skin temperature was warm.

Case 8

Figure 25 shows a seventy year old female with known diabetes for forty years. This is an advanced case of Charcot's disease. There is total destruction of all the articulations of the foot. The patient's only complaints referrable to the foot were numbness, paresthesia and edema.

Case 9

Figure 26 shows Charcot Foot in a patient with spina bifida. The patient was never a diabetic.

Case 10

Figure 27 shows a seventy year old male diabetic maintained on insulin mixtures. There is a draining ulcer at the head of the proximal phalanx of the left hallux. Osteomyelitis is present in the region of the ulcer. Observe the calcified vessel in the first metatarsal interspace. This is an example of differential diagnosis of osteomyelitis versus Charcot joint. A rule that I find helpful in differentiation is that if you can touch bone with a sterile probe in the base of the lesion or in the base of the sinus tract, you are dealing with osteomyelitis.

Case 11

In figures 28–30 the patient is a forty-five year old male diabetic. He has been maintained on oral hypoglycemic agents and diet. Figure 28 is an X-ray of the patient's foot in January 1978. There is an ulcer at site of marker. The patient failed to keep appointments and was not seen again until August 1978. Figure 29 shows a deep ulcer and sinus tract following eight months of neglect. X-ray (Figure 30) with probes in place shows the extent of massive osteomyelitis at the head of the first metatarsal base and the base of the proximal phalanx.

Case 12

The case in Figure 31 illustrates the depth of anesthesia that can occur in a diabetic foot. The patient is a fifty year old female known to have diabetes for twenty years. She has been maintained on N.P.H. insulin and diet. Her chief complaint on examination was painless swelling of the fifth toe. There was no history of trauma. Please observe the fracture of the proximal phalanx. Observe the thinning of the second, third and fourth proximal phalanges.

Case 13

The patient in Figure 32 is a forty-five year old male known to have diabetes for fifteen years. He was treated for an ulcer in the out-patient clinic of a hospital for several months without success. The head of the fifth metatarsal bone was readily seen on examination. Under aseptic conditions the head of the metatarsal was excised. He healed uneventfully in three weeks following this simple surgical procedure. Due to the patient's profound neuropathy, the procedure was carried out without use of local anesthetic. Figure 33 shows the excised head of the fifth metatarsal bone. Figure 34 shows the lesion healed.

REFERENCES

1. Riordan, D.C.: The hand in leprosy. Part II. Orthopedic aspects of leprosy. *J. Bone Jt. Surg.*, **42-A**:684, 1960.

2. Bauman, J.H., Girling, J.P., and Brand, P.W.: Plantar pressures and trophic ulceration. *J. Bone Jt. Surg.*, **45-B**:652, 1963.

3. Schwartz, G.S., Berenyl, M.R., and Siegel, M.W.: Atrophic arthropathy and diabetic neuritis. *Am. J. Roetgenol.*, **106**:523, 1969.

4. Boehm, H.J., Jr.: Diabetic charcot joint. Report of a case and review of the literature. *New Eng. J. Med.*, **267**:185, 1962.

5. Degenhardt, D.P., and Goodwin, M.A.: Neuropathic joints in diabetes. *J. Bone Jt. Surg.*, **42-B**:769, 1960.

6. Peterse, A.: Arthropathia diabetica. *Acta Orthop. Scandinav.*, **30**:217, 1960.

7. Martin, M.M.: Charcot joints in diabetes mellitus. *Proc. Roy. Soc. Med.*, **45**:503, 1952.

8. Knutsson, F.: Diabetic arthropathy. *Acta Radiol.*, **36**:114, 1951.

9. Naide, M., and Schnall, C.: Bone changes in necrosis in diabetes mellitus. *Arch. Intern. Med.*, **107**:380, 1961.

10. Phemister, D.B.: Lesions of bones and joints arising from interruption of the circulation. *J. Mt. Sinai Hosp.*, **15**:55, 1948.

11. Pogonawska, M.J., Collins, L.C., and Dobson, H.L.: Diabetic osteopathy. *Radiology*, **20**:265, 1967.

12. Gondos, B.: Roentgen observations in diabetic osteopathy. *Radiology*, **91**:6, 1968.

13. Sinha, S., Choodappa, S., Munichoodappa, M., and Kozak, G.P.: Neuro-arthropathy (Charcot joints) in diabetes mellitus. *Medicine,* **51**:191, 1972.

CHAPTER 6

Antibiotics

It is becoming increasingly difficult to keep abreast of all the antibiotics available to the podiatrist. The management of foot infections can be more specific. Culture and sensitivity studies, using all the available antibiotics as possible therapeutic agents, have given the podiatrist a valuable modality. Our therapeutic approach can be guided by laboratory findings. The clinical response should still be the ultimate factor in the choice of a therapeutic agent.

Antibiotics can be classified as bacteriostatic, such as the tetracyclines, erythromycin, the sulfonamides and nitrofurantoin. This classification depends on the resistance of the host (patient) to be effective. The patient must have the ability to aid in the localization of the infection, such as increased vascularity in presence of infection and leukocytic diapedesis. Antibiotics classified as bacteriocidal are the penicillins, bacitracin, kanamycin, neomycin and vancomycin. This group of antibiotics are least dependent on host factors to be effective.

Park and Strominger[1] first suggested that penicillin destroyed bacteria by interfering with the cell wall formation through the inhibition of the synthesis of mucopeptide in the cell wall. It is necessary to give high concentrations of the penicillins, ampicillins, methicillins and cephalothin to abruptly halt cell wall synthesis.

In addition to the penicillins, the podiatrist often uses the tetracyclines. This group of antibiotics proves effective only after they have suppressed the protein synthesis of the pathogenic microorganism.[2] Erythromycin, likewise, is effective by inhibiting the protein synthesis. They disturb the ribosomal configuration of the bacteria.[3] The aminoglycoside antibiotics, such as streptomycin, neomycin and gentamicin, destroy bacteria directly by inhibiting the production of protein by the microorganism.

TOXICITY

It is apparent that if the antibiotic can destroy or inhibit the growth of bacteria, it can have deleterious effects upon the patient. While the penicillins are considered the least toxic of the antibiotics, it is not uncommon to find the patient who is allergic to the drug. Deaths have been reported following the use of penicillin. Anaphylactic reactions are not uncommon. It is vital that the podiatrist have in his office agents to offset untoward reactions. Included among the emergency items and measures should be an airway, oxygen, antihistamines, tourniquets, intravenous steroids and epinephrine solution. In addition to anaphylaxis, antibiotics can be hepatotoxic, nephrotoxic, and ototoxic.

Side effects may vary from an elevated body temperature to dermal manifestations ranging from mild morbilliform lesions to overt purpura. Exfoliative dermatitis, erythema multiforme, serum sickness and, as previously mentioned, the much more serious anaphylactic reactions occur. Antifungal agents such as griseofulvin can cause leukeopenia. Broad spectrum antibiotics have been known to decrease the prothrombin levels of the blood with resulting spontaneous bleeding. The normal bacterial flora of the intestinal tract can cause gastrointestinal symptoms. Cross sensitization and overgrowth of pathogenic organisms can occur with any of the known antibiotics. It is abundantly clear that the antibiotics, although life-saving at times, are not a panacea. There is still no substitute for a traumatic debridement of a lesion with sterile instruments in the hands of a competent podiatrist.

Modern podiatry tends to be a "defensive" practice. This is true for modern medicine as well. The art of medicine and the art of podiatry are slowly becoming things of the past. This is due mainly to the growth in the number of attorneys. It is, therefore, imperative that the podiatrist be familiar with the bacterial flora of the normal skin, the bacterial flora of an ulcer and the abraded tissue.

Friedman and Gladstone[4] report the most common organisms in their series of cases were Staphylococcus aureus, Staphylococcus epidermidis, Enterococcus, Proteus mirabilis, E. Coli and Aerobacter aerogens. In addition to the above pathogens, I have cultured the Streptococci, Proteus vulgaris, and Serratia marcescens, as well as fecal anaerobes from lesions of the foot.

Before the culture and sensitivity studies can be reported, 24 to 48 hours have elapsed. It is wise to administer a "broad spectrum" antibiotic in a large enough dosage to allow for a therapeutic blood level to be attained. One must realize that if one is dealing with poorly perfused tissue a much larger dose of antibiotic than would be considered adequate for a normally perfused area must be prescribed.

One should not prescribe any antibiotic until one has done a careful history. The history must include allergy, known sensitivity, renal function, hepatic function and, if possible, the name of any previously administered antibiotic. With the advent of antibiosis a new era was born. The rates of amputation and loss of life have been markedly curtailed. Amputation of a toe should never be done if there is no evidence of sepsis. The surgical amputation of a toe in the diabetic need never be carried out if sepsis is not an overwhelming factor in the clinical picture. Removing a toe is only the precursor to further proximal amputations.

In vitro tests of susceptibility to antimicrobial agents are essential in the management of the diabetic ulcer. One should strive for, and develop, the clinical judgment and acumen necessary to recognize clinically the most efficient antibiotic in any given situation. This is an art that comes only with years of clinical study and mature judgment.

One cannot wait for laboratory findings if the patient has gram negative bacteremia. Sepsis, in this instance, cannot wait for a specific identification of the pathogen. If sepsis is suspected and the pathogenic organism is not immediately identified, it is wise to use a combination of antibiotics. The concurrent use of a penicillinase-resistant penicillin, such as oxacillin, and tobramycin may be indicated. Table 6-1 lists the antibiotics that are felt to be useful for (1) both gram negative and gram positive pathogens, (2) gram positive microorganism only, (3) gram negative microorganisms only, and (4) fungi. Table 6-2 lists the antimicrobial drugs of choice for specific infecting organisms.

THE DIABETIC FOOT

GENERAL NOTES

If the patient is allergic to penicillin, a cephalosporin may be used as an alternative antibiotic. However, one should be aware of the fact that the same patient may be allergic to the cephalosporin. Patients sensitive to penicillin have experienced severe hypersensitivity reactions when treated with a cephalosporin.

Serious adverse or side effects can be encountered with the use of several antibiotics, including clindamycin, vancomycin, chloramphenicol, neomycin, and carbenicillin; therefore, their use should be reserved for fulminating infections only.

Always culture and identify the aerobic and anaerobic bacteria. Remember that the culture and sensitivity tests are not infallible. You can get a clinical response with reduction in the infectious process with an antibiotic that shows minimal growth inhibition of a particular pathogenic organism.

Tetracyclines are not recommended for children and pregnant women. In addition, they are never to be given with meals. Their binding properties are well documented.

If an anaerobic pathogen is cultured from the lesion, the primary therapeutic procedure is debridement. Current literature has shown that hyperbaric oxygen is a most useful adjunct to debridement[5] and massive doses of antibiotics are necessary. Remember, this patient must always be an in-patient of the hospital.

In addition to overt allergic responses, the patient may have such side effects as ototoxicity, neurotoxicity, nephrotoxicity and hepatotoxicity with the use of particular antibiotics.

Gentamicin, tobramycin and amikacin should never be given together with carbenicillin or ticarcillin in the same intravenous drip.

A gentle, aseptic debridement of necrotic tissue is still more effective in controlling necrotic lesions than antibiotics. Antibiotics are adjuncts, and are not to be considered the primary or first line fighters of lesions in the diabetic foot.

Penicillin G is considered by most authorities the antibiotic of choice for all anaerobic infections. The exception to this rule is the infection caused by Bacteroides fragilis, for which chloramphenicol is the antibiotic of choice.

72

ANTIBIOTICS

Table 6-1. Antibiotics Useful for Various Infections

I. General (Gram Positive, Gram Negative) Antimicrobials
Amikacin (Amikin) I.M., I.V.
Amoxicillin (Polymox) P.O.
Ampicillin (Amcill, Omnipen, Penbritin, Polycillin, Principen, Totacillin) P.O.
Cefazolin (Ancef, Kefzol) I.M., I.V.
Cephalexin (Keflex) P.O.
Cephalothin (Keflin) I.V.
Cephradine (Velosef) (Anspor) P.O.
Doxycycline (Vibramycin, Doxy II) P.O.
Tetracycline (Achromycin, Tetracyn, Tetrex, Sumycin) P.O., I.M., I.V.

II. Gram Positive Antimicrobials
Clindamycin (Cleocin) P.O., I.M.
Cloxecillin (Tegopen) P.O.
Dicloxacillin (Dynapen, Pathocil, Versapen) P.O.
Erythromycin (Ilotycin, E-Mycin, Erythrocin, Bristamycin) P.O., I.M., I.V.
Methicillin (Staphcillin) I.M., I.V.
Nafcillin (Unipen) P.O.
Lincomycin (Lincocin) I.M.
Oxacillin (Prostaphlin) P.O., I.M., I.V.
Penicillins
   Benzathine (Bicillin LA) I.M.
   Procaine (Wycillin) I.M.
   Benzathine and G. Procaine (Bicillin CR) I.M.
   Potassium I.M.
   Sodium I.M.
   Potassium (Pen-Vee K, Veetids, V-Cillin K) P.O.
Spectinomycin (Trobicin) I.M., I.V.
Vancomycin (Vancocin) I.V., I.M.

III. Gram Negative Antimicrobials
Carbenicillin (Geocillin, Geopen) P.O., I.M., I.V.
Chloramphenicol (Chloromycetin) P.O., I.M.
Colistimethate (Coly-Mycin) P.O., I.M.
Gentamicin (Garamycin) I.M.
Kanamycin (Kantrex) P.O.
Streptomycin I.M.
Tobramycin (Nebcin) I.M.
Trimethoprim — Sulfamethoxazole (Bactrim, Septra)

IV. Anti-Fungal Agents
Amphotericin B (Fungizone) I.M.
Flucytosine (Ancobon) P.O.
Griseofulvin (Fulvicin) P.O.
Nystatin (Mycostatin) P.O.

Table 6-2. Antimicrobial Drugs of Choice

Infecting Organism	Drug of First Choice	Alternative Drugs
Gram-Positive Cocci		
Staphylococcus aureus		
non-penicillinase producing	penicillin G or V	a cephalosporin, clindamycin, vancomycin
penicillinase producing	cloxacillin, dicloxacillin	cephalosporin, clindamycin, vancomycin
Streptococcus pyogenes (Group A) and Groups C & G	penicillin G or V	an erythromycin
Streptococcus, Group B	penicillin G	chloramphenicol, an erythromycin
Streptococcus, viridans group	penicillin G with or without streptomycin	a cephalosporin, vancomycin
Streptococcus bovis	penicillin G	a cephalosporin, vancomycin
Streptococcus, Enterococcus group, endocarditis or other severe infection	ampicillin or penicillin G with streptomycin, kanamycin or gentamicin	vancomycin with or without streptomycin, kanamycin or gentamicin
uncomplicated urinary tract infection	ampicillin or penicillin G	a tetracycline
Streptococcus, anaerobic	penicillin G	clindamycin, a tetracycline, an erythromycin, chloramphenicol
Gram Positive Bacilli		
Bacillus anthracis (anthrax)	penicillin G	an erythromycin, a tetracycline
Clostridium perfringens (welchii)	penicillin G	chloramphenicol, clindamycin, a tetracycline
Clostridium tetani	penicillin G	a tetracycline, a cephalosporin

Gram Negative Bacilli

Bacteroides	penicillin G	clindamycin, an erythromycin; a tetracycline
Enterobacter	gentamicin or tobramycin	carbenicillin or ticarcillin, kanamycin, chloramphenicol, a tetracycline
Escherichia coli	gentamicin or tobramycin	ampicillin, carbenicillin or ticarcillin, a cephalosporin, kanamycin, amikacin, a tetracycline, trimethoprim-sulfa-methoxazole, chloramphenicol
Proteus mirabilis	ampicillin	gentamicin or tobramycin, carbenicillin or ticarcillin, a cephalosporin, kanamycin, amikacin, trimethoprim-sulfa-methoxazole, chloramphenicol
Other Proteus	gentamicin or tobramycin	carbenicillin or ticarcillin, kanamycin, amikacin, a tetracycline, trimethoprim-sulfamethoxazole, chloramphenicol
Providencia (Proteus inconstans)	amikacin	kanamycin, gentamicin, tobramycin, carbenicillin or ticarcillin, trimethroprim-sulfamethoxazole, chloramphenicol
Serratia	gentamicin or tobramycin	carbenicillin or ticarcillin, kanamycin, amikacin, trimethoprim-sulfamethoxazole, chloramphenicol
Shigella	ampicillin	trimethoprim-sulfamethoxazole, chloramphenicol

Other Gram Negative Bacilli

Acinetobacter (Mima, Herellca)	gentamicin or tobramycin	kanamycin, amikacin, chloramphenicol, minocycline

75

REFERENCES

1. Park, J.T. and Strominger, J.L.: Mode of action of penicillin. *Science,* **125**:99, 1957.

2. Benbough, J.E., and Morrison, G.A.: The molecular basis of an inhibition by tetracyclines. *J. Gen Microbiol.,* **49**:469, 1967.

3. Weinstein, L.: Modes of action of antibiotics on bacteria and man. *N.Y.S. J. Med.,* **66**:2166, 1972.

4. Friedman, S.A., and Gladstone, J.L.: The bacterial flora of peripheral vascular ulcers. *Arch. Dermatology,* **100**:29, 1969.

5. Thomas, C.Y., Grouch, J.A., and Guastello, J.: Hyperbaric oxygen therapy for pyoderma gangrenosum. *Arch. Dermatology,* **110**:445, 1974.

CHAPTER 7

Therapy

The major role played by the podiatrist who treats the diabetic foot is the prevention of gangrene. Bell[1] and others report the documented incidence of gangrene in diabetic men to be over 50 times the incidence in non-diabetic men. The incidence of gangrene in the diabetic female was found to be over 70 times the incidence in the non-diabetic female. These figures were found in the age group over 40.

The literature is replete with theories regarding the etiology and the basic cause of this common life-threatening disease. An accepted concept of the etiological background consists of a triad of factors. Vascular insufficiency, neuropathy and infection appearing in combination in the diabetic patient will result in a gangrenous limb.[2] Vascular insufficiency, perhaps, is the major etiological factor. It is purely academic whether the impaired blood flow on atheromatous plaques that occlude the lumen of a large or small vessel is the causative factor in diabetic gangrene. It is now accepted by those in authority that the problem of diminished vascularity results mainly from the "basement membrane disease", or small vessel disease.

Diabetic neuropathy certainly plays a role in the etiology of a gangrenous lesion. Whenever a patient presents himself with impairment of pain conduction, loss of temperature perception, paresthesia or diminished vibratory sense, it is necessary to rule out diabetes mellitus. The clinical appearance of Charcot Foot on X-ray and clinical observation is discussed in Chapter 6. Suffice it to say at this point that the patient with a neuropathic foot may have excellent pedal pulses, no loss of hair, normal skin turgor, normal temperature and a large necrotic ulcer. One must be aware of the fact that the neurogenic ulcer is painless and the Charcot joint is likewise pain-free.

The growth of bacteria in the traumatized epithelium of the diabetic is well known. The tissues become a fine culture media for the invasion of aerobic, as well as anaerobic, bacteria. The podiatrist must be aware of this fact when ordering culture and sensitivity studies. Louie et al[3] point out that anaerobic bacteria coexisted with aerobic bacteria in 18 out of 20 diabetic ulcers. When a portal of entry has been established, whatever the exciting factor, one can expect to find staphylococci, streptococci, gram negative rods, fungi, and yeast, in addition to the gram negative anaerobes such as Bacteroids fragilis and Bacterroides melainogenicus, and the gram positive anaerobes such as Clostridia perfringes and C. Paraputrificum. A frequent anaerobic bacteria is the gram positive Peptococcus species. The most frequent isolates of the aerobic variety reported by Louie[3] were the Proteus species, enterococci, staphylococcus and Escherichia coli.

The fact that the diabetic ulcer may contain many strains of bacteria which can lead to ascending cellulitis, thrombophlebitis, septicemia, septic shock and death reinforces one of my previous statements. The podiatrist should surround himself with competent medical specialists. If he is caring for the diabetic foot, he must be aware that he cannot and should not attempt to manage the patient independently.

CAUSATIVE FACTORS

Spontaneous Infarctive Lesions

The patient with peripheral arterial occlusive disease develops gangrenous areas in much the same manner as does the patient with arteriosclerotic heart disease. Coronary vessels may spontaneously become occluded, and the area involved may become infarctive, e.g., coronary thrombosis and myocardial infarction. The process is usually slow, insidious and progressive. This same sequence of events occurs in the foot as thrombosis in a local vessel occurring spontaneously and without external influences. The infarctive area, if it involves a small region, is looked upon as a local gangrenous lesion. It is not uncommon to find the first manifestations of sclerotic arterial disease in a local foot infarction. This may be followed days, weeks or months later by myocardial infarction, or these may occur in reverse order.

Embolic disease is another cause of local lesions. However, an embolus in the lower extremity is usually wedged in a vessel proximal to the foot. The resultant clinical picture is more dramatic and acutely fulminating. In the neuropathic foot and its common sequela, Charcot Foot, trophic ulcers are often seen; here again, without external trauma.[4] Possible traumatic factors are listed in Table 7-1.

PRINCIPLES OF THERAPY

It is important to realize that: (1) the lesions appear on the foot in which vascular supply is impaired; (2) the impairment may stem from atherosclerotic disease in the large vessels; (3) while large vessels such as the dorsalis pedis and posterior tibial may be palpable, disease of the basement membrane of the microscopic vessels of the toes may be present; (4) diabetic tissues are more vulnerable to the invasion of pathogenic microorganisms; (5) the diabetic picture may become markedly altered in the presence of infection; and (6) neuropathy.

Table 7-1. Local Trauma Superimposed on Vascular Insufficiency

---

1. Mechanical
   a. Poorly fitting footgear
   b. Stubbing or injuring a toe without being aware of it (neuropathy)
   c. Pressure necrosis from standing still for long periods of time
   d. Mechanical weight of neglected clavi and tylomas
   e. Trauma from the examining clinician (if one exerts enough pressure to blanch patient's nail bed, it is enough to cause necrosis)
2. Chemical
   a. Corn plasters, with invasion of pathogenic microorganisms
3. Thermal (inability of vascular tree to dissipate superficial heat in the presence of neuropathy)
   a. Hot water bottles, radiators, sunlight, heat lamps
   b. Cold temperature exposure, as in frostbite

When ulceration is present, the following measures are employed:

1. Complete bed rest, which is safest and best accomplished by hospitalizing the patient.[4-7] The head, not the foot, of the patient's bed should be elevated approximately 6 inches.

2. Antibiotic sensitivity studies should be done to determine the specific microorganism and the specific medication to be prescribed. Large doses of the specific antibiotic are essential, whether they are given parenterally or orally. It is not unusual to administer up to 20 grams daily of the appropriate antibiotic to a patient with severe occlusive arterial disease and an active infected gangrenous ulcer.

3. No manipulation or trauma to the foot.

4. Debridement under aseptic techniques with no trauma when infection is under control.

5. Use of free volatile, nascent iodine.

6. Consultation for care of the patient's general needs.

7. Arteriography to determine if arterial reconstructive surgery is indicated.[8] Arterial surgery has a definite but limited use in the management of necrotic lesion.[8,9]

8. Since the patient is kept in bed for several weeks, it is necessary that the patient carry out active flexion and extension of the feet to eliminate the complications of phlebothrombosis and stasis edema.

9. When ambulation is allowed, the shoe should be adjusted to prevent weight-bearing on the site of ulceration.[1]

It is not uncommon to find a well-controlled diabetic become a severe diabetic with ketosis in the presence of a seemingly minor infection. Therefore, it becomes the responsibility of the podiatrist to secure competent medical consultation in order that the patient be provided with complete and total care.

Obviously, there is no panacea. Whatever therapy is used, the greatest ally is time. Systemic measures to improve vascularity have been found wanting. Infusion of normal saline solution, popular several years ago, it is not now generally advocated. Intra-arterial infusions of histamine, as suggested by Mufson,[10] have not withstood the test of time. In my experience, parenteral medications, including vasodilators and anticoagulants, have not proved successful.

SURGICAL THERAPY

Angiography is essential in the selection of cases in which surgical intervention may be attempted. Best results are obtained when the presenting complaints are rest pain, neuropathy and ischemic ulceration. Atheromatous infiltration in the femoropopliteal system is best treated by means of autogenous venous bypass grafts.[11] This procedure, as well as endarterectomy, should be attempted only in the presence of a good "run-off" in the distal vessels.

Infrapopliteal arterial occlusive disease is not readily amenable to vascular surgery. Lumbar sympathectomy or its substitute, phenol or alcohol blockage of the lumbar sympathetic chain, have been advocated by some surgeons. While these procedures produce a rise in surface temperature, they seldom influence the course of gangrenous lesions of the foot.

Karmody and Jacobs[12] report that from a series of 86 feet undergoing successful revascularization, only 26 were not subsequently amputated. There is no doubt that vascular surgery plays a part in the salvaging of the diabetic limb in which there has been reduction in blood flow. However, in spite of improvement in surgical technique and the use of microsurgery, the clinical results leave much to be desired.

EXCISION OF METATARSAL HEADS

Lesions on the plantar aspect of the foot overlying the metatarsal heads, in the majority of instances, can be cured by the conservative route. The use of orthotics, shoe adjustments, and plaster of Paris casts play an important part in the management of lesions. When conservative measures fail, then, and only then, one should consider surgical intervention. I have found that the excision of the head of a lesser metatarsal, which in fact is part of the base of the plantar lesion, very often will effect a clinical cure of a recurrent indolent ulceration.

The vascular status, as well as the diabetic control, of the patient must be considered prior to surgical removal of the head of a lesser metatarsal. In this instance, the opinions of the vascular disease specialist and the internist, as well as that of the podiatric surgeon, must be in accord; namely, that the projected result warrants the surgical risk. The podiatric surgeon must be convinced, with reasonable medical certainty, that the surgical procedure is necessary and warranted. This determination can only be made after all conservative means have failed to heal a plantar lesion.

The preferred surgical approach to the metatarsal heads is a dorsal one, but it can also be done through the plantar surface. Meticulous handling of the tissue is of paramount importance throughout the procedure. The podiatric surgeon must be aware of the formation of transfer or new ulcerations that can and do occur adjacent to the original lesion. The use of an orthotic device and the wearing of the correct shoe now become part of the management of the diabetic foot.

MEDICATION AND DRESSING

Local antiseptic measures include the use of all known antibiotics and so-called proteolytic enzymes. Kanof has reported preliminary studies with gold leaf.[13] The local application of gelatin sponge, as reported by Milberg and Tolmach,[14] has a limited use. Many products have been suggested, including powdered dextrose or salicylic acid. However, in my experience, the use of ointments and the like macerates the tissue and further complicates the situation, regardless of the active ingredient. Likewise, in our experience, wet dressings of boric acid and epsom salt macerate tissues when used over a protracted period of time.

The judicious use of hydrogen peroxide as an irrigating solution is helpful. Hydrogen peroxide may be used as an irrigating agent in deep-seated, indolent ulcers. Hydrogen peroxide has been used intra-arterially by Finney et al[15] in the treatment of diabetic ulcers and gangrene. They have successfully used an infusion of 250 ml of a 0.12% solution of hydrogen peroxide in 5% dextrose in water. The infusion is given at the rate of 10 to 20 ml per minute and introduced directly into the superficial femoral artery. They have reported a series of 45 patients with excellent results, including a reduction in the thickness of the capillary basement membrane in the treated extremity as compared to the non-treated limb, which served as a control. Further evaluation is necessary before any firm conclusions can be drawn. I have found the use of porcine grafts of limited value (see Figures 35–37). The use of gentian violet, brilliant green and other dyes is of no value. They simply mask the clinical picture and have no therapeutic value. I have found that the "proteolytic enzymes" have no place in the management of the diabetic ulcer. The use of povidone-iodine (Betadine®) has minimal application. Hyperbaric oxygen therapy has been reported as a useful adjunct in the management of the diabetic ulcer and gangrene. It is effective in spite of the absence of anaerobic organisms.[16] Treatment usually involves exposure in a hyperbaric chamber at 2 atmospheres for 30 minutes daily for seven days. The exposure to hyperbaric oxygen varies with each institution. There is no one accepted treatment plan or exposure time. It can vary from 30 minutes per day to six to eight hours per day for a five day period. This practice is followed by a one week rest period and, depending upon the response, the patient is again exposed to hyperbaric oxygen.

In deep-seated lesions, I have found the use of a polymer of dextran (Debrisan®) a most useful adjunct. Used with debridement, drains, and an iodine solution, it serves a useful function

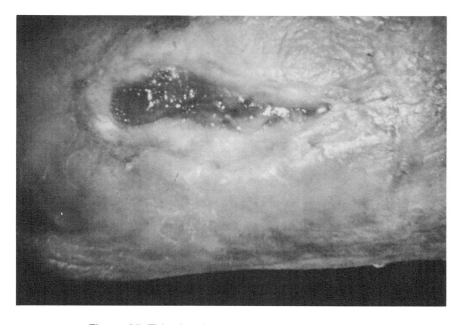

Figure 35. This ulcer is treated with a porcine graft.

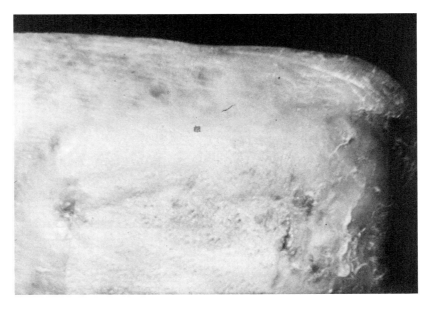

Figure 36. Porcine graft in place.

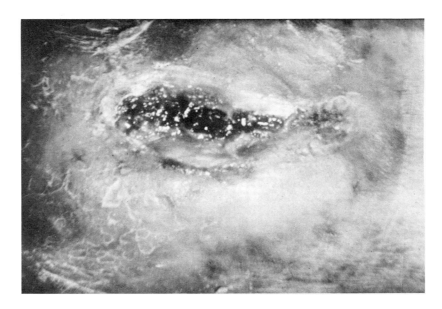

Figure 37. One week after graft. The base of the ulcer is healthy; however, epithelium has not developed.

and makes a definite contribution to the management of the diabetic ulcer. I find little value in using the polymer of dextran in the superficial ulceration. In fact, in two cases the lesions deteriorated.

The use of vasodilators in the management of ischemic ulcers has little or no value. If the lesion is caused primarily by vasospasm there may be a place for its use. However, I find little evidence to support the notion that an arteriosclerotic vessel can be made to increase the size of its lumen.

The antiseptic properties of the halogens have been known for years; however, methods of application had been found wanting until Collens et al[5] published their work, in which a method for the release of nascent, volatile iodine was described. This method of treatment is as satisfactory today as it was when the paper was presented in 1962. Briefly, the solution is prepared by dissolving 0.5 grams of potassium iodide in 100 ml of water, to which 1.0 gram of iodine crystals is added. The iodine solution, by virtue of the low vapor tension of the solution, releases free volatile iodine very quickly. Approximately 0.4 grams of the iodine goes into the solution, so that there is a supersaturated solution, with the crystal iodine entering the solution as the free tri-iodide complex leaves the medium. This unstable compound provides a rapid and continuous release of free nascent iodine.[9]

The solution can be used in any of several ways and in a combination of dressings. Sinus tracts may be loosely packed and the iodine solution placed directly on the drain. The tri-iodide solution may be applied directly to the slough, or it may be placed upon a sterile gauze pad which is then sandwiched between two dry sterile gauze pads and incorporated into one dressing (see Figures 38–43).

In the acute phase, as stated previously, the patient should be hospitalized and allowed no walking privileges. Dressings should be changed daily. As the clinical picture improves, as evidenced by reduction in edema, relief of cellulitis, demarcation of the lesion and appearance of granulation tissue, the dressings may be changed every other day. It is important to remember that the slough will separate spontaneously. Only at this point should instrumentation be undertaken to facilitate, and possibly shorten, the period of disability. Liquefaction necrosis or separation of the dry mummified lesion are excellent prognostic signs. One should never attempt to debride when the gangrenous patch is immobile.

Liquefaction at the line of demarcation will allow the gangrene to be mobile. Only then should it be debrided.

Human amniotic membrane may in the future prove to be a useful adjunct in the management of gangrenous ulcers of the feet. Gruss and Hirsch[17] report a series of 120 patients in which they found that human amniotic membrane serves as a useful biologic dressing in traumatic and nontraumatic wounds. This should prompt further investigation in the area of diabetic ulceration and gangrene.

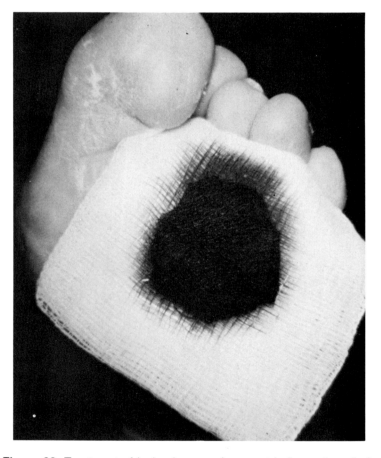

Figure 38. Treatment of lesion by use of nascent iodine not applied directly to skin. A 4 x 4 sterile gauze pad is placed on the foot, then a 2 x 2 sterile gauze pad saturated with nascent iodine is placed overlying the lesion.

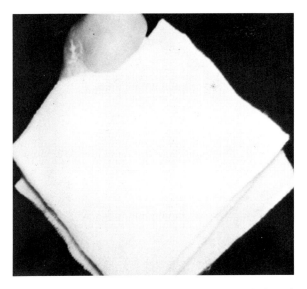

Figure 39. Same patient, with dry sterile gauze pad placed over nascent iodine pad.

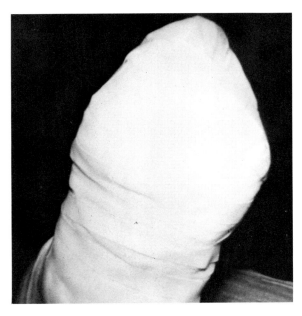

Figure 40. The dry pad and the pad soaked in nascent iodine are held in place by a sterile bandage.

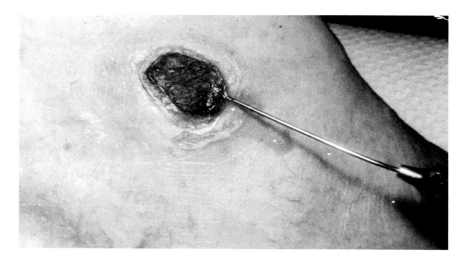

Figure 41. Irrigation of gangrenous lesion with nascent iodine solution. Note: the lesion is irrigated and viable tissue is never injected. The patient is a seventy year old diabetic. The diabetes is controlled with 20 units of protamine zinc insulin per day. The lesion followed the trauma of poorly fitting shoes. The patient received oral antibiotics in keeping with culture and sensitivity studies in appropriate doses.

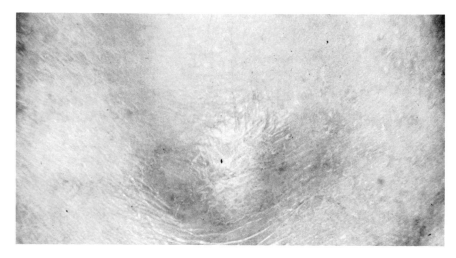

Figure 42. Lesion completely healed after two months of local care. Therapy involved (1) local application of nascent iodine three times per week, and (2) penicillin 500 mg every 6 hours orally.

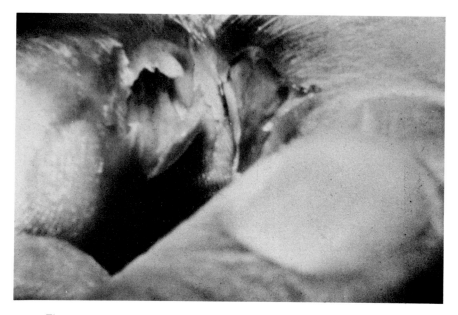

Figure 43. Tincture of iodine is known to cause chemical burns. The patient, thinking I had applied tincture of iodine in a previous year for therapy of an interdigital ulcer, treated himself. The result was an iodine burn. Tincture of iodine is *not* the weak iodine *solution* described in the text.

SHOE MODIFICATION FOR AMBULATION

Alterations in footgear are necessary to permit minimum weight-bearing. Bauman et al[18] have reported an extensive study of plantar pressure in the trophic foot. They have shown that continuous pressure of only slight magnitude is enough to deprive tissue of its blood supply. If this continuous pressure is maintained for a length of time, ischemic necrosis occurs. Kosiak[19] and Lindan[20] demonstrated, in animal experiments, that this pressure need only be 0.08 kg/cm^2. If we assume that total ischemia is produced when external pressure is greater than systolic blood pressure, it can be computed that 0.2 kg/cm^2 is sufficient to produce necrosis. If a patient stood completely still for a sufficiently long period of time, he could develop gangrene on the plantar aspect of the foot. This would be particularly so in the patient with peripheral vascular disease, with or without diabetes.

The shoe must be remodeled to provide a tread surface proximal to the lesion, or distal to the lesion in the case of heel lesions. The use of latex devices, foam rubber wells and adjusted molded appliances serves very well to relieve pressure at sites of healed lesions. A pressure grid and plaster of Paris casts are necessary to prepare a proper appliance. Redistribution and relief of pressure areas are necessary to prevent recurrences.

SOME GENERAL CONSIDERATIONS

All diabetic patients must have a careful history and vascular evaluation before any measures can be instituted. Ischemia and hypoxia are the common complications that result in serious sequelae and delay in healing. Diabetics with fair blood flow can have extensive necrotic lesions. Trophic lesions are common in the diabetic patient with neuropathy. Patients in this category experience reduced pain or, in some cases, no pain at all when trauma has occurred.

The podiatrist familiar with this disease sees evidence of capillary fragility with resulting subungual and subcutaneous hematomas. I concur strongly with Black and Whitehouse[21] that callus, once formed on the foot, must be trimmed aseptically at least once a month. This will prevent necrosis and infection that occur when calluses and calvi are neglected and allowed to grow into heavy masses of hyperkeratotic tissue. The same frequent meticulous care is necessary for onychogryphotic and onychomycotic nails.

Dryness of the skin, notably in the heel region, is the cause of heel fissures. The patient must be advised as to proper, strict foot hygiene, in addition to the application of an emollient ointment.

Diabetic patients must be alerted to the importance of proper footgear in cold weather as well as in warm weather. Exposure to extreme temperatures, whether cold or hot, should be avoided at all costs. The feet of these patients must never be exposed to direct sunlight or direct or indirect heat and cold.

The modern podiatrist, trained in basic medical fundamentals and armed with professional judgment and experience, plays a vital part in the health of the nation. While it is important to recognize the local lesion, it is equally imperative that a general physician or medical specialist work in close cooperation with the foot doctor. For the sake of the patient, the podiatrist and medical practitioner must work together as a team.

Modification of shoes to allow for ambulation for the patient with lesions on the plantar aspect of the foot can be very frustrating. The basic principle in designing such modifications is to prevent weight-bearing at the site of the ulcer. There are certain pitfalls to be avoided. There should never be sharp edges, whether the material is made initially of leather or plastic. One must make full use of material such as foam rubber, sponge rubber, plastazote and plastic material for shoe inlays (Figures 44–49).

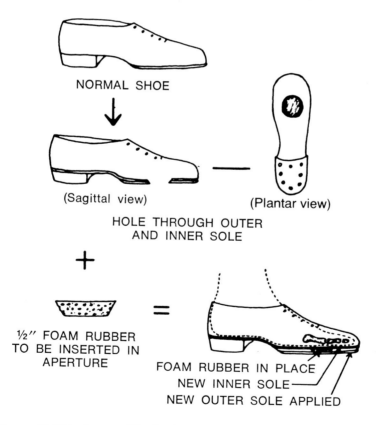

NORMAL SHOE

(Sagittal view)　(Plantar view)

HOLE THROUGH OUTER
AND INNER SOLE

+

½″ FOAM RUBBER
TO BE INSERTED IN
APERTURE

=

FOAM RUBBER IN PLACE
NEW INNER SOLE
NEW OUTER SOLE APPLIED

Figure 44. This shoe modification is to be used only after a lesion on the plantar aspect of the foot has healed.

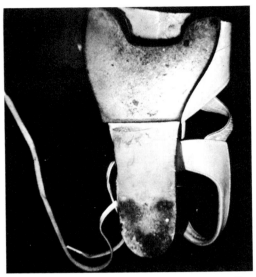

Figure 45. Shoe modification in the shape of a U. This allows for ambulation when the lesion is at the heads of metatarsals number 3 or 4. It is important to line the insole with foam rubber sufficiently thick to prevent pressure at the edges of the U-shaped cut-out. The outer sole of the shoe should be one inch thick.

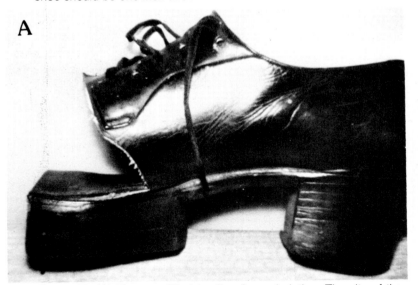

Figure 46. (A) Shoe modified to allow for ambulation. The site of the ulcer is the anterior of the foot or toes. (B and C) Shoe modified to allow ambulation for a lesion of the heel. Observe the placing of one-half inch thick foam rubber at the edge. The edge should be bevelled. This will prevent pressure at the sharp leather end of the insole.

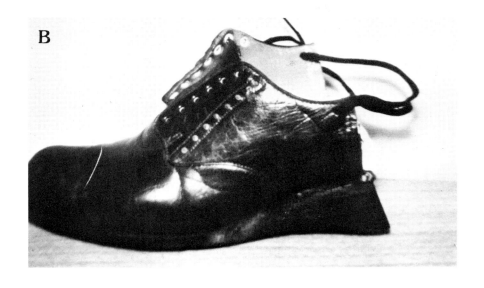

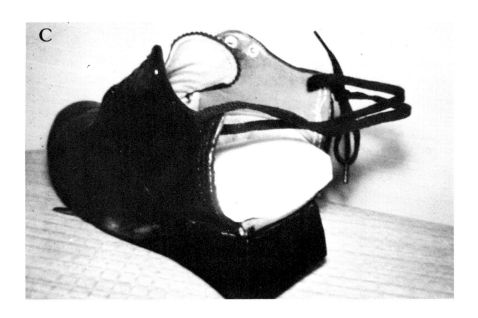

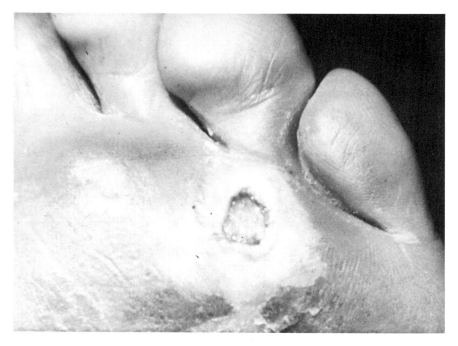

Figure 47. Lesion on plantar aspect, at the head of the fourth metatarsal. This patient is a sixty year old male diabetic receiving regular protamine insulin. The patient failed to respond to usual therapy due to the fact that he was walking, despite orders to the contrary.

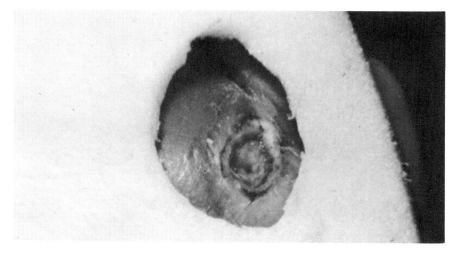

Figure 48. Plastazote insole with aperture in place.

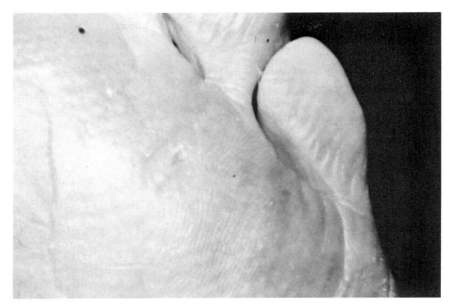

Figure 49. Lesion completely healed using appropriate antibiotic, control of diabetes and suitable appliance for relief of weight-bearing.

SUMMARY

There have been many illusions and misconceptions with regard to determining the adequate vascularity, management and therapy of diabetic ulcers. It is important to keep the following points in mind:

1. A patient may have both a palpable pedal pulse and frank gangrene of the foot. While this is not the usual finding, one practicing this branch of medicine should be well aware of the fact that this can occur.

2. Allowing the patient to walk with an open lesion, without adequate protection, in order to improve their "blood supply" is an order fraught with danger. The patient with an open lesion on the plantar aspect of the foot should not be allowed to walk.

3. It is a fallacy to use "capillary return" as an indication of arterial supply. This is physiologically unsound.

4. The presence of hair on the foot does not mean the patient has a good blood supply and, therefore, cannot develop gangrene.

I have seen many cases in which the patient has hair on the foot and also has gangrene of the toes.

5. To allow the patient to have edema in the presence of an open lesion is physiologically unsound. The presence of edema is never a good prognostic sign.

6. The use of whirlpool baths and similar physical modalities is of no use and can, indeed, be detrimental in management of the diabetic foot.

With the addition of the ever-increasing number of antibiotics, the practitioner has been given more time to treat the patient conservatively. There is no one best method in the treatment of the diabetic ulcer. I fully agree with Robson and Edstrom,[22] conservative management of the diabetic ulcer is the method of choice. Conservative care has never resulted in a greater number of amputations. Quite to the contrary,[23] conservative management of the diabetic ulcer and gangrene has markedly reduced the number of amputations, and, in the rare instance when amputation is necessary as a life-saving procedure, the level of amputation is more distal than one could or would predict at the outset.

REFERENCES

1. Bell, E.T.: Atherosclerotic gangrene of the lower extremities in diabetics and non-diabetic persons, *Am. J. Clin. Pathol.,* **28**:27, 1957.

2. Ellenberg, M.: Diabetic foot. *N.Y. J. Med.,* **73**:2778, 1973.

3. Louie, T.J., et al: Aerobic and anaerobic bacteria in the diabetic foot ulcers. *Ann. Intern. Med.,* **85**:461, 1976.

4. Leving, M.E.: Diabetes mellitus as manifested in the foot. *J.A.P.A.,* **56**:49, 1966.

5. Collens, W.S., and Rakow, R.B.: Conservative management of gangrene in the diabetic patient. *J.A.M.A.,* **181**:692, 1962.

6. Karbelnig, M.J.: The diabetic foot. *Med. Sci.,* **8**:94, 1966.

7. Root, H.F.: Pre-operative medical care of the diabetic patient. *Postgrad. Med. J.,* **40**:120, 1966.

8. Haimovici, H.: Femoral arteriography. *J. Cardiovase. Surg.,* **8**:1, 1964.

9. Frank, E.D.: Peripheral arterial disease. *Med. Sci.,* **9**:581, 1961.

10. Mufson, I.: Peripheral vascular diseases and their care. *J.A.M.A.,* **155**:815, 1954.

11. Shatz, I.J.: The chronically ischemic lower limb. *J.A.M.A.*, **197**:915, 1966.

12. Karmody, A.M., et al: Salvage of the diabetic foot by vascular reconstruction. *Orthop. Clin. N. Amer.*, **7**:957, 1976.

13. Kanof, N.M.: Gold leaf in the treatment of cutaneous ulcers. *J. Invest. Derm.*, **43**:441, 1964.

14. Milberg, I.L. and Tolmach, J.A.: Treatment of chronic leg ulcers with absorbable gelatin sponge (Gelfoam) powder. *J.A.M.A.*, **156**:12, 1954.

15. Finney, J.W., Lynn, J.A., Jay, B.E., et al: *Treatment of Refractory Ischemic Ulcers in Humans by Regional Hyperoxia (Intra-arterial Hydrogen Peroxide)*, Institute for Biomedical Research Baylor University Medical Center, Dallas, Texas, 1976.

16. Thomas, C.Y., Grouch, J.A., and Guastello, J.: Hyperbaric oxygen therapy for pyoderma gangrenosum. *Arch. Dermatology*, **110**:445, 1974.

17. Gruss, J.S., and Hirsch, D.W.: *Canad. Med. Assoc. J.* **118**:1237, 1978.

18. Bauman, J.H., Girling, J.P., and Brand, P.W.: Plantar pressures and trophic ulceration. *J. Bone J. Surg.*, **45B**:652, 1963.

19. Kosiak, M.: Etiology of decubitus ulcers. *Arch. Phys. Med.*, **42**:19, 1961.

20. Lindan, O.: Etiology of decubitus ulcers. *Arch. Phys. Med.*, **42**:774, 1961.

21. Black, M.A., and Whitehouse, F.W.: Place of conservatism in the medical and surgical management of foot complications in the diabetic. *Med. Digest*, **6**:211, 1966.

22. Robson, M.C., and Edstrom, L.E.: Conservative management of the ulcerated diabetic foot. *Plast. Recon. Surg.*, **59**:551, 1977.

23. Rakow, R.B.: The treatment of necrotic lesions in the diabetic patient. *J.A.P.A.*, **57**:412, 1967.

CHAPTER 8

FOOT SURGERY

I have stated previously that diabetes mellitus is a constitutional disease. The management of all aspects of the disease should be controlled by the qualified internist.

Foot surgery, as it applies to the diabetic patient, must be considered and judged to be of major importance. When evaluating a podiatric surgical case, the podiatrist must keep in mind two important factors: (1) the vascularity of the foot should be within normal limits, and (2) the diabetes should be controlled.

As a general rule it is unwise and unsafe to perform surgery on the foot of a diabetic for cosmetic reasons. Surgery of the foot should be restricted to only those patients with intractable pain. All conservative means should be attempted before one contemplates surgical intervention in the diabetic patient. It is unsafe and unwise to attempt to do any surgical procedure on the diabetic in one's office. All diabetic foot surgery should be performed in a hospital, and then only after the proper medical work-up and medical clearance are obtained. The trauma from any surgery, however minimal, can elevate the blood glucose. It is not the unusual case wherein a controlled diabetic is converted to an uncontrolled diabetic following so-called minor surgical procedures.

HAZARDS DURING SURGERY

The podiatrist must be aware of the following hazards during surgery.

(1) The risk of hypoglycemia is greater during surgical proce-

dures if the surgery is not performed with an intravenous dextrose infusion. Hypoglycemia may mask neurogenic shock (see Table 8-1, "Insulin Shock").

(2) If the procedure is to be done under local anesthesia, it is safer to use regional block. It is unwise to infiltrate the base of the toe or any area of the foot with local anesthesia. The mere presence of an increased intracellular pressure may cause tissue necrosis. Under no circumstances should epinephrine be used with the local anesthetic solution. The vasoconstriction can produce a gangrenous toe, if injected into the base of a digit.

(3) Avoid the use of tourniquets. A constricting band, interrupting the blood flow, can cause necrosis of tissue in the diabetic foot. One must keep in mind that the basement membrane of the capillaries is a very delicate microscopic structure that is easily traumatized and rarely recovers from mechanical trauma.

(4) Do not over-sedate the patient. The elderly patient is unpredictable with regard to effective sedation. Minimal doses are the rule. It is not uncommon to find the elderly patient in an excited state when, after sedation, one would expect the opposite.

(5) Deaths have been reported from cerebral vascular accidents, myocardial infarction, and renal shut-down, as well as from generalized sepsis. Taking a good history is of paramount importance prior to surgery of any patient. A patient may deny that he or she is a diabetic. It is helpful to know the background of the patient as well as his or her presenting complaints.

Diabetes mellitus is an inherited disease. A double recessive genetic disease may effect 25% of the offspring. It is, therefore, incumbent upon the podiatrist to elicit a history of diseases such as diabetes and ask whether siblings and/or parents have had the disease. It is important to realize that the patient may have inherited the double recessive gene for diabetes; however, the date he develops the disease can be influenced by such exciting causes as surgical trauma.

The patient may have a normal blood sugar and give a history of several stillbirths or several infants born weighing over 10 pounds. If this is the case, the podiatric surgeon should be aware that he has a latent diabetic under his care. It is likewise the case if the patient gives a history of neuropathy, proteinuria, repeated urinary tract infections, retinopathy, polyuria, polydypsia, polyphagia, pruritis vulvae and/or loss of weight.

PRE- AND POSTOPERATIVE MANAGEMENT
OF THE DIABETIC

Preoperative Work-up

All diabetic patients undergoing foot surgery should be admitted to the hospital two days prior to the scheduled surgery. On admission, the podiatrist should examine both lower extremities. The vascular supply and the neurological evaluation of the patient must be recorded on the patient's chart. An electrocardiogram and chest X-ray should be done on the patient, and their interpretation should be made a part of the hospital record. A complete blood count, as well as a complete urinalysis, must be documented. A Sequential Multiple Analyser (SMA 12) is a good screening profile, and should be ordered for every patient. This procedure will give the values for calcium, inorganic phosphorous, glucose, urea nitrogen, uric acid, cholesterol, total protein, albumin, total bilirubin, alkaline phosphatase, lactic dehydrogenase (LDH), and glutamic-oxalacetic transaminase (SGOT). If the patient is to have general anesthesia, it is wise to obtain the preoperative values for the electrolytes, namely, potassium, sodium, chloride and carbon dioxide. The renal function should be monitored for two days prior to surgery. It is, therefore, necessary to order blood urea nitrogen (BUN) for two consecutive preoperative days.

Preoperative Orders for the Diabetic Having
Local Block Anesthesia

In the diabetic patient controlled under this heading there is no change in his oral or insulin quality or quantity. On the night prior to surgery, it is prudent to give the patient a mild sedative upon retiring. Those commonly prescribed are the short-acting barbituates, such as pentabarbital (Nembutal®), secobarbital (Seconal®), or thiopental (Pentothal®) in appropriate dosage. A good rule to follow is that the sedative dose is one-third the hypnotic dose, or, in other words, the hypnotic dose is three times the sedative dose. One hour before surgery it is advisable to order morphine sulphate (15 mg) or Demerol® (75 mg) given subcutaneously. A ten minute betadine scrub after shaving all pedal hair, followed by draping the leg in sterile towels, is carried out in the

101

patient's room the night before surgery. This preoperative scrub does not eliminate the usual and customary preoperative scrub and painting on the operating table.

Postoperative Orders for the Diabetic Having Local Block Anesthesia

The diabetic diet consisting of 150 grams of carbohydrate, 75 grams of protein and 50 grams of fat is ordered. It is wise to increase the protein intake by 25 grams for the two immediately postoperative days. This increase in protein, furnishing an additional 100 calories, is usually well tolerated without altering the anti-diabetic agent. It is not wise to allow the patient to ambulate for the first 12 hours. In extensive procedures, this may be extended to the first one or two postoperative days. A mild analgesic is in order. I have found codeine sulphate (15 to 30 mg) an ideal drug. It causes little or no lethargy and enables the patient to eat. The urine is to be tested for glucose and acetone at each voiding (fractional urines). The fasting blood sugar should be done each morning before breakfast.

Preoperative Orders for the Diabetic Having General Anesthesia

The patient should be admitted for his preoperative work-up two to three days prior to the scheduled surgery. The results of the patient's electrocardiogram and chest X-ray must be documented. It is essential that he have a fasting blood sugar for two preoperative days. It is likewise essential that the blood urea nitrogen be determined each morning for the two preoperative days. An evaluation of the peripheral blood flow, as well as a complete neurological examination, should be part of the hospital chart. All of the work-up and pertinent medical and podiatric history must be part of the chart.

It is important that the patient be denied any food or fluids by mouth after 9 P.M. on the eve of surgery (N.P.O.). The apprehensive patient may be given a short-acting barbituate intramuscularly upon retiring. The preoperative medication is left to the anesthesiologist. His orders usually call for morphine sulphate, 15 mg (gr. 1/4) plus atropine or scopolamine 0.4 mg (1/150 gr.) given in separate injections intramuscularly on call to the operating room.

No insulin or oral agent (tolbutamide or any sulfaureas) is given the night before the surgery or when calling the patient to the operating room.

It is important to prevent dehydration, furnish the necessary fluids and promote homeostasis. It is, therefore, important to start an intravenous drip of 5% glucose in one liter of normal saline. This intravenous load should only be administered to the young patient. The elderly can be easily overloaded. Hypervolemia can result. The elderly should receive 250 ml of 20% glucose in slow intravenous drip (25 drops per minute). It is important to add regular insulin at this time to the management of the patient. This may be ordered by the internist in the form of 15 to 35 units of regular insulin subcutaneously. The insulin may be added to the intravenous infusion.

Postoperative Orders for the Diabetic Having General Anesthesia

It is vital to monitor the glucose and carbon dioxide combining in the blood, as well as to monitor the urine for glucose and acetone immediately after surgery. It is wise to keep the intravenous going until the patient retains two meals. This will prevent dehydration and hypoglycemia in the event that the patient vomits his first or second oral feeding. Fractional urines must be noted. Insulin coverage is as follows: If the patient is spilling 1 plus glycosuria, no insulin is necessary. If the patient is spilling 2 plus glucose, 5 units of regular insulin are given subcutaneously. If the patient is spilling 3 plus glucose, 10 units of regular insulin are given subcutaneously. If the patient is spilling 4 plus glucose, 15 units of regular insulin are given subcutaneously. For every plus of acetone, add five units of regular insulin. The complication of ketosis is not uncommon and must be dealt with vigorously and immediately. Never over-sedate the patient. I have found codeine, 15 to 20 mg given by mouth, if the patient is able to retain oral medication, a competent analgesic. It is of little importance which analgesic is ordered, provided that the minimal doses are given. The patient is not allowed bathroom privileges for the first 48 hours. The diet should consist of 1500 to 1700 calories (200 grams of carbohydrate, 80 grams of protein and 40 grams of fat). If the patient does not void spontaneously, he should be catheterized every eight hours.

RECOGNITION OF HYPOGLYCEMIA
AND HYPERGLYCEMIA

It is important for the podiatric surgeon to recognize and differentiate insulin shock (hypoglycemia) from insulin coma (hyperglycemia). Tables 8-1 and 8-2 will serve as a guide to the recognition of shock and coma.

GLUCOSE TOLERANCE TEST

If there is any question about whether the patient is diabetic or not, it is wise to perform a glucose tolerance test. Figure 50 is a

Table 8-1. Insulin Shock (Hypoglycemia)	
Onset	In hours or minutes
History	No dietary indiscretion
	Normal or subnormal temperature
	No infection
	No polydipsia
	No polyuria
	No vomiting except with gastric disturbances
	Taking insulin
	No abdominal pain except with gastrointestinal disturbance
Clinical Signs	Normal hydration
	Skin moist
	Skin pallid or normal
	Normal breathing
	May have convulsions
	Positive neurological signs
	No acetone breath
Laboratory Signs	Urine sugar-free in second voided or catheterized specimen
	No ketonuria
	Hypoglycemia
	Normal CO_2 combining power
	Blood count normal
Response to Glucose Therapy	Rapid Improvement

graph of the normal patient and the diabetic patient. As you will note, the blood is initially drawn on a fasting stomach and then a bolus of 100 grams of glucose is given. The podiatrist who accepts the responsibility of treating the diabetic foot must be aware that there are medications he may prescribe that can have adverse effects on the glucose level of the blood (Table 8-3). Table 8-4 is an outline that will help screen those patients subject to elective surgery; if the patient falls within the normal ranges, surgery may be attempted. For his general fund of knowledge, the podiatrist should be aware of the normal ranges of the chemical constituents of the blood. Table 8-5 sets forth these normal ranges and those conditions that will increase or decrease these constituents.

Table 8-2. Diabetic Coma (Hyperglycemia)

Onset	In days
History	Dietary indiscretion
	Fever
	Infection
	Polydipsia
	Polyuria
	Vomiting
	No insulin taken
	May have abdominal pains
Clinical Signs	Dehydration-soft eyeballs, loss of skin turgor
	Skin dry
	Skin flushed or normal
	Kussmaul breathing
	No convulsions
	Negative neurological signs
	Acetone breath.
Laboratory Signs	Glycosuria
	Ketonuria
	Hyperglycemia
	Low plasma CO_2 combining power
	Leucocytosis and polynucleosis
Response to Glucose Therapy	None

Table 8-3. Factors That Can Effect The Blood Glucose Levels

Drug	Increase Blood Glucose	Decrease Blood Glucose
Analgesic and Anti-inflammatory		
Aspirin and Salicylates		X
Indomethacin	X	
Oxphenbutazone		X
Phenylbutazone		X
Antibiotics and Antibacterials		
Sulfonamides		X
Chloramphenicol		X
Diuretics		
Thiazides	X	
Sedatives		
Barbiturates		X
Stimulants		
Caffeine	X	
Vasoactive Agents		
Epinephrine (Adrenalin)	X	
Tranquillizers and Antidepressants		
MAO inhibitors		X
Chlorpromazine	X	
Miscellaneous		
Probenecid		X
Nicotinic acid (high dose)	X	
Alcohol		X
Nicotine	X	
Pyribenzamine		X
Other Factors		
Arthritis	X	
Coffee	X	
Gastrectomy	X	
Hypertension	X	
Nephritis	X	
Obesity	X	
Prolonged inactivity	X	
Smoking	X	
Strenuous exercise		X
Stress		
Emotional	X	
Fever		X
Infection	X	
Physical		X
Pregnancy	X	
Surgery		X

	Value which would make elective surgery contra-indicated	
Normal Range	**Low**	**High**
RBC: men 4.5 million–6.0 million	3.5	6.5
women 4.3 million–5.5 million	3.0	6.0
Hb: men 14–18 GMS	10	19
women 12–18 GMS	10	18
Hematocrit: men 38–54%	32	52
women 36–47%	32	52
Platelets: 200,000–500,000	100,000	800,000
Bleeding Time: 1–4 min (Ivy)	—	5′
1–3 min (Duke)	—	5′
Coagulation Time: 6–10 min (Lee-White)	—	14′
Capillary Blood 2–4 min (Capil. Tube)	—	—
Sedimentation Rate		
Wintrobe: men 0–6.5 mm	—	—
women 0–15 mm	—	—
Westergren: men 0–15 mm	—	35 m
women 0–20 mm	—	35 m
WBC: 5,000-10,000 per cu mm	4,000	30,000
Juvenile neutrophiles: 3.5%	—	—
Segmented neutrophiles: 54 - 62%	35%	—
Eosinophiles: 1 - 3%	—	10%
Basophiles: 0 - 1%	—	5%
Lymphocytes: 25 - 33%	—	65%
Monocytes: 3 - 8%	—	20%

Table 8-4.

Table 8-5. Commonly Used Blood Tests

	Normal Range	Increased	Decreased
Albumin	6—8 grams/100 ml	Dehydration	Nephrosis Nephritis Burns Congestive heart failure Starvation
Calcium	9-11 mb/100 ml	Multiple myeloma Sarcoma Hyperparathyroidism Bone resorption	Vitamin D deficiency
Chloride	350–370 mg/100 ml	Dehydration	Infections Diarrhea Marked edema Polyuria
Cholesterol	150–300 mg/100 ml	Diabetes Hypothroidism	Anemia Steroid Therapy
Creatine	0.5–0.95 mg/100 ml	Rheumatoid arthritis Diabetes Renal disease	
Creatine Phosphokinase	0-12 Sigma Units/ml	Any muscle injury (myocardial or striated)	

Table 8-5. Commonly Used Blood Tests

	Normal Range	Increased	Decreased
C-Reactive Protein	0	Rheumatic fever Rheumatoid arthritis Myocardial infarction	Steroids
Glucose	90–120 mg/100 ml	Diabetes mellitus Acromegaly Pheochromocytoma Excess steroids Hyperthyroidism	Hepatic disease Addison's disease
Lactic Dehydrogenase	200–650 units/ml	Carcinoma Myocardial infarction Renal and hepatic disease	
Alkaline Phosphatase	1.5–4 (BU) 30–70 (SMA)	Osseous and liver disease (Bone: heat labile, liver: heat stable)	
Phosphorus	2.5–4.5 mg/100 ml	Paget's disease Myeloma	Diabetes
Potassium	3.5–5.1 mEq/L	Acute renal failure	Stress states
Urea Nitrogen	10–20 mg/100 ml	Diabetes Renal and congestive heart failure	
Uric Acid	2.8–6 mg/100 ml	Gout	Salicylate therapy

This table is to serve only as a reference to the most widely used tests in podiatry. The compounds and elements listed are the most commonly affected in the diabetic patient. It is not intended to serve as the sole reference to the blood chemistry available to the podiatrist.

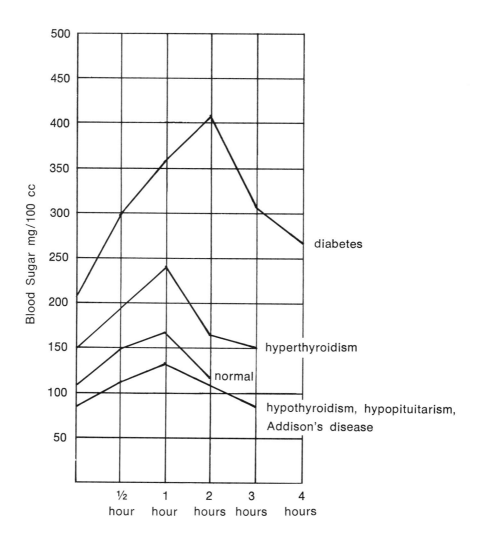

Figure 50. Evaluation of glucose tolerance test.

CHAPTER 9

Patient Instructions and
Contributory Negligence

INSTRUCTIONS TO THE DIABETIC IN THE
CARE OF HIS FEET

Prevention, wherever possible, is to be desired. The diabetic patient can reduce his morbidity and lessen his suffering by adhering to several basic principles. First, he should never walk barefooted; this rule applies to any and all situations. Second, the diabetic must bathe his feet daily in tepid water. The temperature of the water is to be verified as tepid by a member of his or her family who is not a diabetic. Third, he must pat dry his feet and not simply walk away from his bath. Fourth, he must wear properly fitting shoes and stockings. In cold climates, it is advisable for the diabetic to wear woolen socks without elastic bands and fleece-lined shoes. This rule applies to women as well as men. Fifth, if the feet tend to be dry, he should be instructed to gently massage hydrous lanolin into his feet daily. Care must be given to the heel area. This is the site for fissure formation in the dry, cold foot. Fissures are, in fact, linear areas of necrosis. Nails should be cared for by a qualified podiatrist. If the patient has been instructed to use an emery board or commercial product for the reduction of hyperkeratoses, the best and only advice he can receive is to change his physician. The modern physician realizes his responsibility and is not threatened by referral to a podiatrist.

The diabetic should never expose his feet to direct sunlight. Both the feet and legs should be covered with a thick towel if sunbathing is his wish. There is no known physical modality capable of restoring an impaired vascularity. Likewise, there are no known physiotherapy procedures which can reverse the neuropathic, osseous changes and any degenerative process with which the diabetic foot can be afflicted. They are to be condemned both from medical and moral principles. The use of heating devices such as lamps and diathermy can be harmful to the diabetic foot. The diabetic is to avoid this type of therapy for two very important reasons. First, he does not feel extremes of hot and cold (neuropathy). Second, he does not have the vasodilatation necessary to dispel the local application of any modality purported to be of therapeutic value by the creation of heat. Thermal burns and necrosis are well known following the use of this type of physiotherapy.

Foreign bodies imbedded in the inner soles of shoes have been known to cause gangrenous ulcers. It is, therefore, important to inspect the entire inner sole for rough bodies like nails, pins, buttons and pebbles.

The patient should report to his podiatrist any change in the appearance of his feet, or any sudden onset of coldness. Edema, elevation of skin temperature, rubor, cyanosis and pain are not normal signs or symptoms.

CONTRIBUTORY NEGLIGENCE ON THE PART OF THE PATIENT

Contributory negligence on the part of the diabetic patient in the formation of a lesion can either be overt or covert. We all recognize the patient who will take an oath that he or she never walks barefooted. Upon examination, the plantar aspects of the feet are encrusted with bits of paper, particles of sand and strands of hair.

The patient and his family either forget or refuse to remember self-inflicted trauma. I can recall seeing a patient leave my office. He entered his daughter's car. I watched his daughter close the car door on the patient's foot. The next day I received a call from the daughter asking what I did to turn her father's foot "black". Reminding her of her "accident" promptly deflated a situation that had all the earmarks of at least a subpoena.

The use of home remedies and taking the advice of well-meaning friends contribute to the formation of many lesions in the diabetic foot. I have seen a case where acupuncture was used to "cure arthritis". It was too bad that the therapist inserted the needles into a foot that had minimal blood flow. Despite all heroic measures, the patient lost the limb.

The use of stylish shoes plays a major role in the etiology of lesions in the diabetic foot. Just as a snug molded shoe can produce pressure necrosis and gangrene, so too can the high-heeled pointed toe shoe. It is not uncommon to see an ulcer on the dorsum of any toe, although the fifth toe is prone to such a lesion, on the patient insisting on wearing shoes too small for her feet.

The podiatrist may manage a case of an ulcer in the diabetic foot flawlessly. The end result can be a poor one for any reason. The most common negligence on the part of the patient is failure to remain off his feet. The foot doctor's conception of total bed rest and the patient's idea are two very different things.

Taking prescribed medication in ordered doses can be a problem. Cooperation from the family with regard to caring for the patient includes giving medication. All too often this becomes too burdensome for the devoted children. Again, we find contributory negligence on the part of the patient.

The use of "over-the-counter" appliances contributes to the morbidity of the diabetic foot. It is not uncommon to hear that the patient bought a pair of arches from a vendor. The podiatrist is burdened with the task of clearing up a plantar ulceration.

It is human nature to try to place the burden of responsibility upon someone. The diabetic will "cheat" on his diet, forget to take his insulin and do a host of other suicidal machinations. He will tend to blame everyone but the right one, himself.

CHAPTER 10

Care of the Diabetic Foot in Children

The onset of diabetes in children follows a well recognized course. This usually involves a sudden increase in appetite (polyphagia), which may go on for months before polyuria and polydypsia become evident. It is not infrequent to hear a parent say, "My child is on the toilet urinating and at the same time he is drinking water." Following weeks of polydypsia and polyphagia, the child will lose weight, become listless and lose stamina. It is not uncommon, at this point, for the child to complain of nocturnal claudication. As podiatrists, we should be acutely aware of this syndrome. The blood usually shows marked hyperglycemia and the urine is plus 4 for glucose and plus 4 for acetone. It is strictly a problem for an internist with special training in the care of the juvenile diabetic. It is interesting to note that within a short period of time (two to four weeks) with insulin and diet the patient goes into an apparent remission. In fact, it is not unusual to have the patient go into a period of hypoglycemia immediately preceding the period of remission.

On the other hand, the patient may be a brittle or labile diabetic during puberty. Brittleness, as defined by Molnar,[1] is a syndrome of excessive insulin sensitivity and ketosis proneness manifested by extreme and unexplained short-term fluctuations in the parameters of the disease.

Infections will disturb the diabetic balance in a child with great rapidity. Therefore, it becomes a serious clinical problem when we find a paronychia in a diabetic child. It is never to be considered a minor problem. The attending internist must be advised accordingly and immediately. The affected toe is treated in the following manner. The toe is "wet dressed" for 24 hours. It is of little importance just which wet dressing the podiatrist recommends. I find normal saline wet dressing just as efficacious as any solutions. The prime consideration is to keep the child in bed and keep the dressing wet. A broad-spectrum is given by mouth. The dosage will depend on the age and the weight of the child.

Young's Rule: $\dfrac{\text{Age of child}}{\text{Age plus 12}} \times \text{Adult dose} = \text{Child's dose.}$

or Clark's Rule: $\dfrac{\text{Weight of Child}}{150} \times \text{Adult dose} = \text{Child's dose}$

Either of these rules will prove helpful in determining dosage. After twenty-four hours of wet dressings and antibiotics, the spicule of ingrowing toe nail can be painlessly removed. Upon removal of the segment of nail, there is the usual purulent exudate. This should be cultured and sensitivity studies made. The shoe should have the toe box removed. A suitable antibiotic dressing is applied. The dressing is changed every 24 hours. During the phase of active infection, the diabetes may become completely out of control. It is apparent at this point that in order for control of the hyperglycemia and possible ketosis, the internist must adjust the insulin coverage and the diet may be altered.

It is not uncommon to find dermatophytosis and atopic eczema in the diabetic child. As with the adult, a potassium hydroxide-treated scraping of the epidermis should be carried out. If a fungus is present, it usually responds to applications of clotrimazole (Lotrimin®). Atopic eczema often responds to twice daily application of 3% iodochlorhydroxyquin (Vioform®).

Verruca plantaris is not commonly seen in diabetic children. When they occur, however, the treatment of choice is chemical cautery at weekly intervals. A fresh application of 60% salicylic acid ointment and padding of the part will result in a cure in from four to six weeks, depending on the size and location of the verruca.

Diabetic children, like all children, tend to run barefooted and do not bathe frequently. It must be impressed upon the parents of the child that preventive podiatry is very important. Foot hygiene is an integral part of this practice.

The diabetic child is not immune to any of the mechanical deformities seen in the foot. It is possible to have, and with the same frequency as the general population, mechanical malpositioning as subtalar varus or valgus. It is possible to have forefoot varus or forefoot valgus. Tibial torsion is, likewise, seen in the diabetic child.

The rule of thumb in selecting a plan of therapy for this group of children is to never cause impingement on the skin or cause any undue pressure on any point on the foot or leg. It is important to make sure that the shoe accepting the child's foot and the orthotic device are compatible. There is no objection to the use of metal appliances, provided that they fit correctly and are examined with frequent and regular intervals. The child quickly outgrows the orthotic. It is rare for the orthotic to fit correctly after one year's use.

A word of caution is in order. Before the foot specialist makes the decision that the clinical picture and subjective complaints are due to mechanical malformation, *rule out systemic disease.* Rheumatoid arthritis gives protean symptomology. The subjective picture can mimic and mask mechanical deformity. Never assume that because the child is a diabetic, he or she is being carefully monitored. If the child complains of vague pain in the foot or leg and has obvious foot deformities, it does not mean that the child's complaints are caused by the foot defect. The child needs a sedimentation rate, complete blood count, LDH, SGOT, and SGPT, as well as an electrocardiogram. It is only after all these tests are found to be within normal limits that the podiatrist can assume that the child's complaints are a direct effect of the obvious foot defect or malposition.

REFERENCE

1. Molnar, G.D.: Observations on the etiology and therapy of brittle diabetes. *Canad. Med. Assoc. J.,* **90**: 953, 1964.

CHAPTER 11

Lesions on the Foot Other Than Gangrenous Ulcers

Malignant lesions occur on the foot. Many times one mistakes a benign ulcer for a carcinoma. Malignant melanoma, amelanotic melanoma, basal cell carcinoma, squamous cell carcinoma, as well as Kaposi's sarcoma, have been reported on the feet of the diabetic patient. We all are aware of the fulminating malignant course of melanoma. Mitotic neoplasms all metastasize. The obvious difference is the rate of the metatasis. Basal cell carcinoma has the least virulence vis-a-vis metastasizing. The following cases will exemplify the fact that the podiatrist is often the physician who makes the diagnosis. The cases listed were treated for a benign skin pathology by doctors of medicine as well as doctors of podiatric medicine.

Case 1

The patient in Figure 51 is a sixty-seven year old known diabetic for twenty years. He had been treated for one year by several doctors of medicine as well as doctors of podiatric medicine for a fungus condition of his left great toe. Clinical diagnosis of squamous cell carcinoma was confirmed at the time I amputated the hallux. The patient was followed by his internist for six years until evidence of hepatic metastasis was noted.

Case 2

Figure 52 shows a seventy year old male diabetic for twenty years, who presented himself for treatment of an ulcer, plantar

119

aspect of the left foot. The ulcer was present for two years and at no time was it healed. Treatment elsewhere consisted of total in bed care, short leg walking cast and massive doses of antibiotics. An incisional biopsy was performed by me to confirm the clinical diagnosis of squamous cell carcinoma. The entire plantar aspect of the foot was excised and a skin graft from the left thigh was used as a replacement. The skin graft failed. A below-the-knee amputation was performed two and one-half months after the diagnosis was made. The patient was alive for 15 years after the amputation with no evidence of metastasis.

Case 3

Figure 53 shows a sixty-nine year old female diabetic for forty years. She presented herself for treatment of "callus at the distal end of the right toe". The clinical impression was that we were dealing with a sarcoma; the entire mass was excised. The pathology report indicated Kaposi's sarcoma. The patient healed with primary union and to date is well and shows no evidence of other lesions anywhere on the body.

Case 4

The patient in Figure 54 is a sixty-three year old male. He is a known diabetic for twenty years. At the present time his diabetes is controlled by diet alone. For the past three months he has been under the care of his physician for what was diagnosed as "warty growth". On examination, the plantar aspect of the right foot presented a well circumscribed, dark mass, with little or no pigmentation. The mass was painless on walking and palpitation. The surrounding epithelium was normal in appearance. The dressing consisted of a "band-aid". Surgical excision and biopsy was advised and carried out 48 hours after his initial visit. The pathologist's diagnosis was malignant melanoma.

Surgical follow-up: resection of the plantar aspect of the foot extending to the plantar fascia. A skin graft was employed to close the defect. The inguinal nodes were excised and were found to be negative for mitotic figures. The patient has made a satisfactory recovery. It is now 15 months since the excisional biopsy. The patient is free of symptoms at this time.

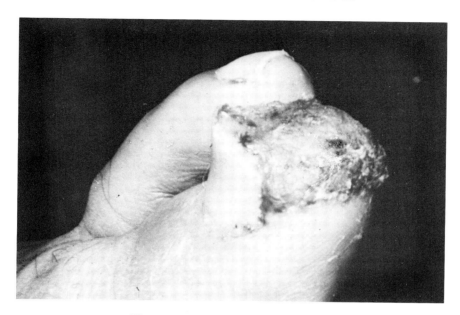

Figure 51. Squamous cell carcinoma.

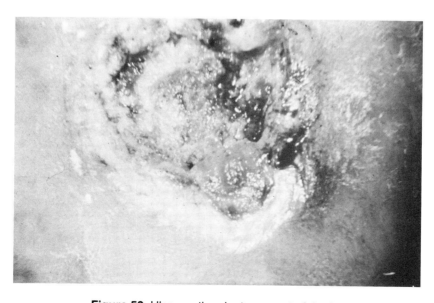

Figure 52. Ulcer on the plantar aspect of the foot.

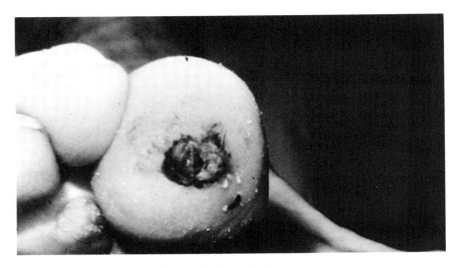

Figure 53. Kaposi's Sarcoma.

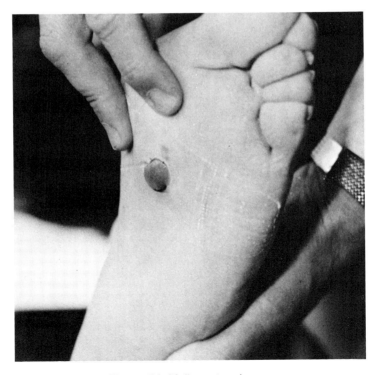

Figure 54. Malignant melanoma.

Case 5

Figure 55 shows a lesion at the plantar aspect of the foot of a forty year old male diabetic. Ulcer did not heal by usual means; excision biopsy showed it to be a benign area of granulation tissue with no evidence of mitotic activity.

Case 6

The patient is a sixty year old female diabetic. Her diabetes was discovered twenty years ago and is controlled by diet alone (Figures 56 and 57).

One month before presenting herself for treatment, she noticed the great toe nail of the left hallux suddenly become "loose". There is no history of trauma, self treatment or iatrogenic influence.

On examination, a segment of nail plate 0.5 cm × 0.75 cm was found attached to the bed and posterior eponichium. The nail bed was wet, with areas of necrosis and pigmentation. The toe was free of pain. The skin was warm, normal turgor and obviously adequately perfused. The pedal pulses were present. Oscillometric readings were within normal limits. Vibrometry was normal and intact. Fasting blood sugar was 125 mg per 100 ml. The blood urea nitrogen was 22 mg per 100 ml. The blood count was within normal limits. The bleeding time was normal, as was the total blood platelet picture.

A clinical diagnosis of melanoma (sub-ungual) was made. An incisional biopsy was performed and a diagnosis of melanoma was confirmed. The depth of invasion, in keeping with Clark's classification, was Level III. An amputation of the great toe was carried out with lymph node resection.

The incidence of lymph node metatases for Level III invasion is approximately 7%. This patient did not have positive lymph nodes. The correlation between Clark's level of invasion and survival after surgery is indicated by the fact that 88% of the patients with Level III invasion are alive after five years.

Case 7

It is obvious to all clinicians well versed in the care of ulcerations of the diabetic foot that not all ulcers are benign. The following is an example.

The patient is a seventy-five year old female (Figures 58 and 59). She had been treated for a "stubborn" ulcer on the plantar aspect of the foot at the head of the second metatarsal phalangeal articulation by her family podiatrist and physician before presenting herself for evaluation. The dorsalis pedis and posterior tibial pulses were absent. Oscillometric readings were reduced bilaterally. The venous filling time was within normal limits. All serology and blood chemistries were within normal limits except for a mildly elevated blood glucose (128 mg %). The lesion appeared as a well demarcated ulcer with an unhealthy, necrotic base. The base, however, was highly vascular and bled easily when a dull probe was used to determine the undermining of the margins. A clinical diagnosis of melanoma was made and the entire lesion excised with normal epidermis at all borders. The lesion was excised to the level of the subcutaneous adipose tissue.

The pathologist's report was malignant melanoma, Level IV. There is a higher percentage of metastases at Level IV than Level III. The patient with Level IV or V should be treated by wide excision and lymph node dissection.

Case 8

Necrobiosis lipoidica diabeticorum (Oppenheim-Urbach disease) is a peculiar diabetic dermatosis (Figure 60). It may appear as a single dermal lesion or it may appear as a pair. They may coalesce and occur in the young diabetic. The area effected is commonly the anterior of the leg. The lesions are well demarcated and circumscribed. There is a loss of the elastic and connective tissue of the skin.

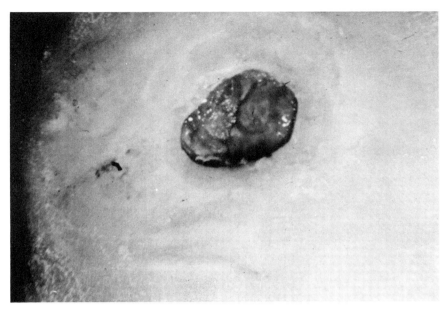

Figure 55. Benign ulcer.

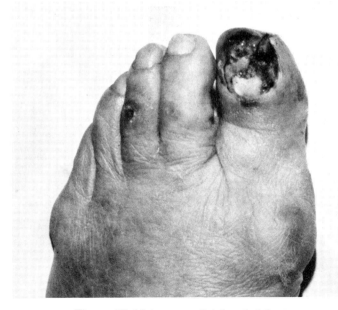

Figure 56. Melanoma, distal end of the toe.

125

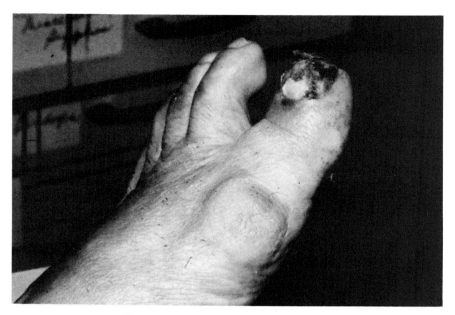

Figure 57. Same patient as Figure 56.

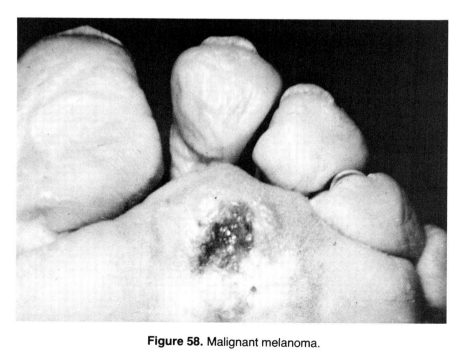

Figure 58. Malignant melanoma.

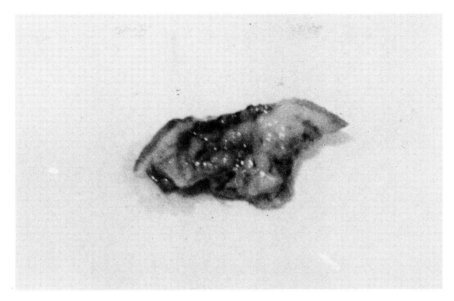

Figure 59. Melanoma excised.

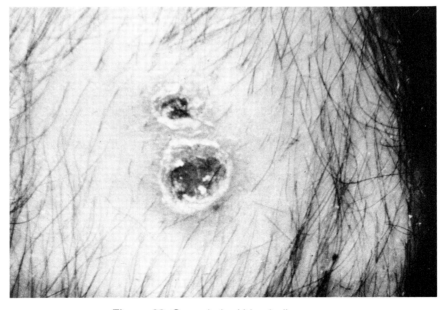

Figure 60. Oppenheim-Urbach disease.

CHAPTER 12

Thermal Gangrene

The diabetic, in spite of good management and proper instructions with regard to his feet, will actually burn his feet. The following two cases will serve as examples.

Case 1

Mr. A.H. is an example of thermal gangrene in a diabetic with severe neuropathic changes. He is a sixty year old male having had diabetes mellitus for thirty years. He has always been controlled with varying doses of daily injected insulin. In spite of weight control and exacting care with regard to his hyperglycemia, he developed a peripheral neuropathy to such a degree that he could not feel his foot literally frying. Vibratory sense was absent in both feet. Oscillometric readings were reduced in both feet. Position sense reduced in both great toes. Sharp and dull sensations were markedly diminished in both feet. Venous filling time was 25 seconds in both feet. Pedal pulses were absent.

In an attempt to warm his feet on a radiator he smelled something burning. Again, I repeat, he felt no pain. Figure 61 shows a burn of the medial aspect of the heel. At this point, he was given a broad spectrum antibiotic and ordered to bed. Dry, local dressings were applied. Three weeks later, Figure 62 shows a well demarcated area of dry gangrene. The eschar was firmly attached to the underlying tissue and no attempt at debridement was made. I would like to emphasize that no attempt at surgical debridement, or any type of manipulation, should be attempted before spontaneous separation takes place. Liquefaction takes place at the margins of the gangrene. Before this occurs, all measures to control

129

infection are employed. So-called proteolytic enzymes are worthless. Attempts to remove the firm, necrotic tissue by a surgeon, general practitioner or podiatrist prematurely result in a catastrophe. Likewise, rough handling of the part by anyone can result in a progression of the necrosis with the loss of a limb.

Figure 63 shows a segment of the eschar removed. This was accomplished with a minimum of trauma. Throughout the management, the patient had culture and sensitivity studies and was given appropriate antibiotics in massive therapeutic doses. The most important aspect in the management of the lesion, other than sterility and minimal trauma, is choosing the proper time for debridement. The proper time is when the eschar becomes mobile. This is an indication that the lesion is undergoing liquefaction at its base. In order words, the foot is now attempting to spontaneously rid itself of the gangrenous patch.

Figure 64 is the same foot with the entire gangrenous patch debrided. The patient is now allowed to walk only with a shoe that has been modified to prevent pressure at the site of the ulcer. At this point, the dressings are changed every third day. This patient was dressed with weak iodine solution. The oral antibiotics, which were given in keeping with the culture and sensitivity studies, can gradually be cut down.

Figure 65 is four months after the thermal burn. The patient is now completely ambulatory and the lesion is healed.

Case 2

The patient is a sixty year old male with known diabetes for twenty years. During a cold night, he attempted to warm his feet on a radiator. The result, shown in Figure 66, is a thermal gangrene. The patient, due to his severe neuropathy, did not feel his foot being burned. Figure 67 was taken six weeks after the trauma.

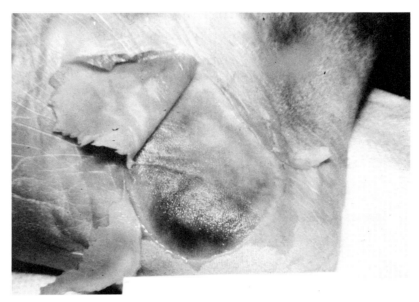

Figure 61. Thermal gangrene.

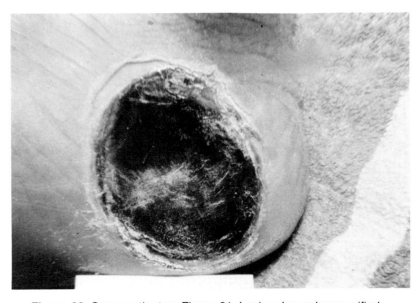

Figure 62. Same patient as Figure 61. Lesion dry and mummified.

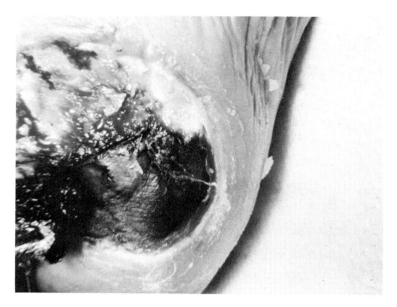

Figure 63. Debridement of dry, mummified, mobile lesion.

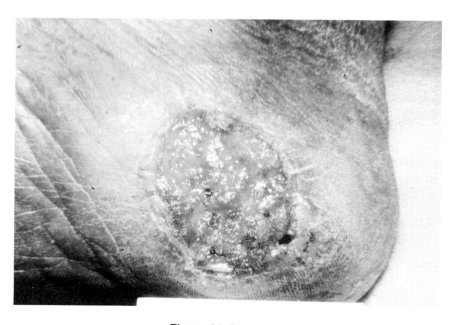

Figure 64. Base of ulcer.

132

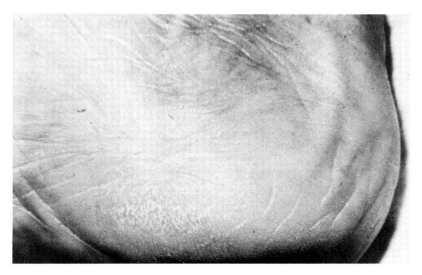

Figure 65. Thermal gangrenous ulcer healed.

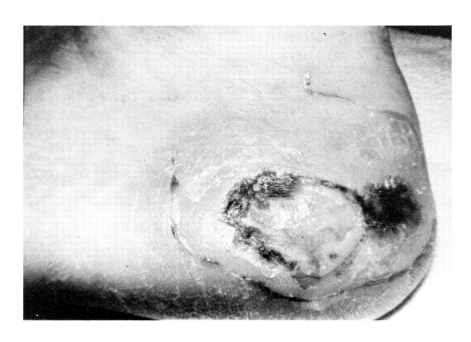

Figure 66. Thermal gangrene.

133

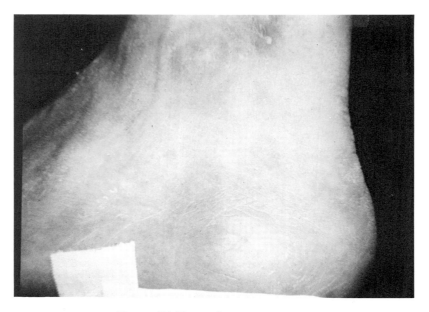

Figure 67. Thermal gangrene healed.

CHAPTER 13

Gangrenous Lesions

Gangrenous lesions and ulcerations can occur anywhere on the foot. The exciting factors can be trauma, chemical or thermal burns, or spontaneous infarction. Many times the etiology can never be pinpointed. The podiatrist must first recognize the fact that the patient has a gangrenous lesion. Secondly, he must do a complete vascular and neurological examination in addition to a careful and meticulous history. The treatment plan calls for complete bed rest, which is best accomplished by hospitalizing the patient, in addition to the following measures. Culture and sensitivity studies must be done for the identification of pathogenic bacteria and antibiotic. The antibiotic of choice should be administered in massive doses. The greater the vascular impairment, the greater the dose of antibiotic. With the patient in the hospital, it is always more efficient to give the antibiotic by the intravenous route. The renal and hepatic system must be monitored daily if the patient is receiving massive intravenous therapy. Locally, the gangrenous area should not be traumatized or manipulated. The use of local antibiotics should be limited to only those which are known to be effective. The use of electric lamps under a cradle is useless and extremely hazardous. The use of physiotherapy is useless. This includes hydrotherapy and all types of electrotherapy.

During the acute phase, at which time the vital signs are monitored every other day, there can be no hard and fast rule with regard to changing dressings. The podiatrist must see the patient as frequently as the clinical picture dictates. As pointed out in the preface, the podiatrist should always have the internist share the responsibility of managing the patient. The vascular surgeon should, likewise, be a member of the health team.

THE DIABETIC FOOT

Case 1

Patient is a seventy year old white, obese female, weighing 180 pounds.

Chief complaint: Massive gangrenous lesion of the right foot.

Present illness: Patient has had gangrene of the right foot, with partial amputation of the great toe some three months before coming under observation. Family refused suggested mid-leg amputation at another hospital.

Past history: Patient is a known diabetic for 20 years and was maintained on protamine zinc insulin (30 units daily before breakfast). The patient has suffered a coronary thrombosis ten years before coming under observation.

System history: Blood pressure was 184/110. All pedal pulses were absent on palpation. The femoral pulses were weak bilaterally. Oscillometric readings were zero below both knees and at both ankles. The patient was hospitalized and consultation with the cardiologist and family physician was obtained throughout the term of care.

Laboratory findings: Urinalysis on admission was 4+ for glucose, 1+ for albumin, negative for acetone, CBC was within normal limits. The fasting blood sugar was 180 mg. The blood urea nitrogen was 35 mg, serum cholesterol 260 mg %. The electrolyte studies were within normal limits. Repeated cultures from the lesion showed staphylococcus albus, coagulase negative. Antibiotic sensitivity showed chloramphenicol, penicillin, erythromycin and neomycin as antibiotics of choice. EKG tracing showed evidence of old myocardial infarction.

Diagnosis: Acute infectious gangrene, peripheral arteriosclerosis obliterans, arteriosclerotic heart disease, diabetes mellitus and hypertension (Figure 68).

Course in hospital: The patient was allowed no bathroom privileges for her entire 34 days of hospitalization. A suitable diabetic diet, low in cholesterol, was ordered. Her insulin dose was ordered by the family physician and varied between 40 and 60 units of protamine insulin daily. She received chloramphenicol (500 mg q6h). The white count was checked periodically for signs of depression in WBC. None was found at any time, nor any evidence of blood dyscrasia encountered. The lesion was dressed daily. Dressings consisted of irrigation of the necrotic mass with a solution of tri-iodide complex and chloramphenicol. Debridement, aseptically, and without trauma, was carried out at the bedside as often as deemed necessary.

Home Care: The same regimen was followed while the patient was at home. After two months of intensive care, she was able to have bathroom privileges with a properly cut shoe. She was discharged, healed, one year after coming under care (Figure 69).

Case 2

A fifty-nine year old male presented himself for treatment of his left great toe.

Chief complaint: Gangrenous lesion of the left great toe and region of the head of the left first metatarsal bone (Figure 70).

Exciting factor: Patient stated he "was breaking in a new shoe and developed a blister on his foot."

Past History: Patient is a known diabetic for 15 years. Paresthesia and numbness of both feet past several years. His diabetes has been maintained with diet and 20 units Lente insulin per day.

Positive physical findings: A ruptured bleb on the medial aspect of the left great toe. An intact bleb overlying the medial aspect of the head of the first metatarsal bone. Pedal pulses were unobtainable.

System history: Evidence of hypertensive heart disease, anginal syndrome and orthopnea were elicited.

Physical findings: Blood pressure on admission to hospital: 200/110; oscillometric readings: 1½ below knees and 0 above both ankles.

Laboratory findings: Cholesterol: 230 mg; B.U.N.: 21 mg; F.B.S.: 128 mg; W.B.C.: 8,900; differential within normal limits. Hemoglobin: 13.2 grams; urine: negative for glucose, acetone and albumin. Electrolytes and total proteins were within limits.

Diagnosis: Diabetes mellitus, peripheral arteriosclerosis, two gangrenous patches on the left foot.

Course in hospital: Medical management and cardiac status under supervision and direct control of internist. The patient received erythromycin, 500 mg p.o. = q.6h., as dictated by antibiotic sensitivity studies of the exudate. Insulin requirements were directed by consultant internist. Lesion was irrigated with tri-iodide solution daily for the three weeks during which the patient was hospitalized. When he was allowed to return home, his shoe was adjusted to allow for ambulation without weight-bearing. The patient was discharged as cured four months after initial treatment (Figure 71).

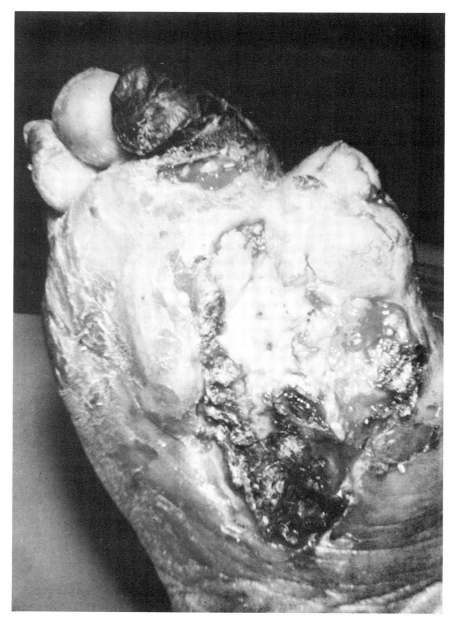

Figure 68. Massive gangrene, wet and dry.

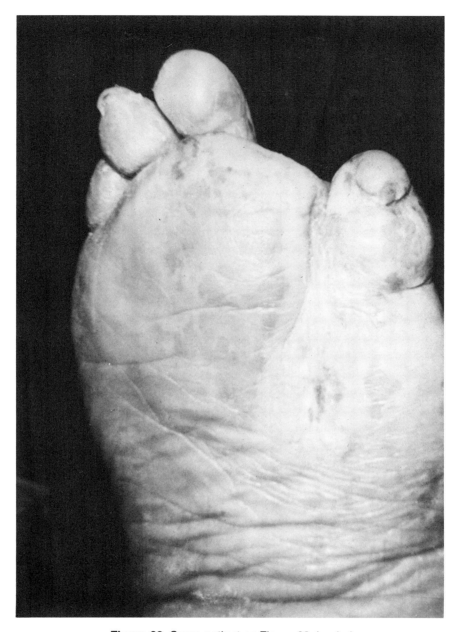

Figure 69. Same patient as Figure 68, healed.

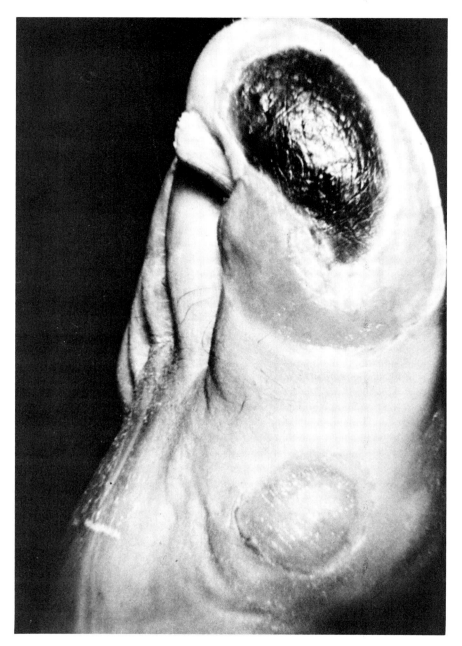

Figure 70. Trauma from shoe.

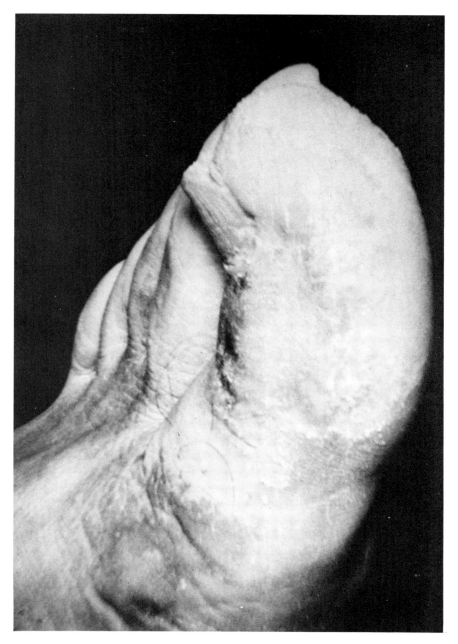

Figure 71. Trauma healed.

Case 3

Patient is a sixty-two year old male. He is a known diabetic for ten years.

Present illness: The patient has had an ulcer on the medial aspect of the left hallux. He was under the care of his internist for six months prior to consultation (Figure 72).

System history: Blood pressure was 190/96. All pedal pulses were absent. Venous filling time was thirty seconds, bilaterally. Both feet are cold with poor skin turgor. Fasting blood sugar was 210 mg per 100 ml.

Laboratory studies: SMA 12 was within normal limits, except for the hyperglycemia. Urinalysis on the initial visit was 3+ for glucose, negative for albumin and negative for acetone. Culture and sensitivity studies revealed staphylococcus albus, coagulase negative. Antibiotic of choice was erythromycin.

Course: The patient was ordered to remain at home, in bed. He received erythromycin, 250 mg four times a day. His foot was dressed with nascent iodine solution daily. Debridement was done every seven days. The lesion was totally healed in two weeks. He was fitted with a latex jacket to remove weight-bearing. He has been free of ulceration for the past two years (Figure 73).

Case 4

Recurrent ulcer, plantar aspect of foot overlying third metatarsal head. Ulcers in this area do very well if one respects the head of the underlying metatarsal bone (Figure 74). However, if the blood supply to the foot is inadequate, surgery is contraindicated. This patient did very well with conservative management. Bed rest, culture and sensitivity, appropriate antibiotics and nascent iodine proved effective. In the sub-acute stage, the patient was allowed limited ambulation with a shoe modified to remove any pressure on the ulceration. The ulcer healed in seven weeks (Figure 75). The patient has remained free of ulceration for two years wearing a leather and cork appliance in his shoe designed to relieve the site of the previous ulcer from weight-bearing.

Case 5

Similar lesion to Case 2. In this case, however, the ulcer ex-

142

tended to, and included, the medial sesamoid bone (Figure 76). This was removed, in the office, without untoward complications. Here too, the patient did very well with appropriate antibiotics and local application of nascent iodine solution. Figure 77 was taken the same day as Figure 76, showing medial sesamoid excised. Figure 78 was taken seven weeks later.

Case 6

This is a two hundred fifty pound male diabetic with a history of ulceration on the plantar aspect of the foot overlying the fifth metatarsal head (Figure 79). The head of the metatarsal was excised through the sinus tract on the plantar aspect of the foot. The approach to the involved metatarsal head is dictated by the course of the sinus tract. One merely follows the direction of the tract when excising the bone. Here again, anesthesia is unnecessary due to severe diabetic neuropathy.

Follow-up therapy: the sinus tract is loosely packed with sterile gauze and the area flushed with nascent iodine solution. Figure 80 shows the foot healed eight weeks later.

Case 7

The patient is a diabetic with a large abscess on the dorsum of the foot. The course of therapy, as outlined in the text, produced a most gratifying result. As you will note, one can readily see the dorsal tendons exposed in the base of the lesion (Figure 81). Figure 82 shows the foot healed after eight weeks of treatment.

Case 8

The patient has been a known diabetic for fifteen years. The vascular supply to the foot is poor. One must be ever on the alert for spontaneous infarctive gangrene. This case is typical. The patient gives no history of trauma. The lesion at the outset looks benign. In several days, however, a rapid downhill course ensues. Figure 83 was taken five days before Figure 84. Figure 85 was taken three months later. Here again, the course of therapy is explained in detail within text.

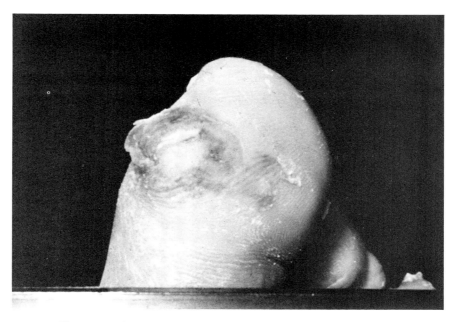

Figure 72. Gangrenous ulcer that had been treated as a callus.

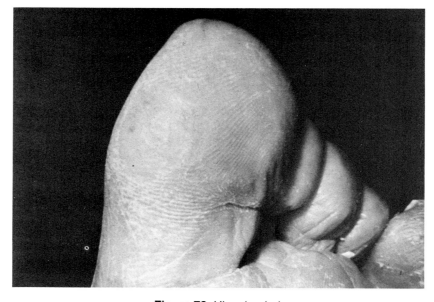

Figure 73. Ulcer healed.

144

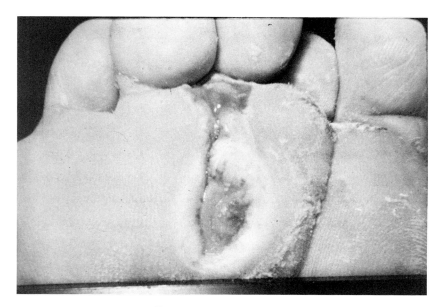

Figure 74. Recurrent ulcer.

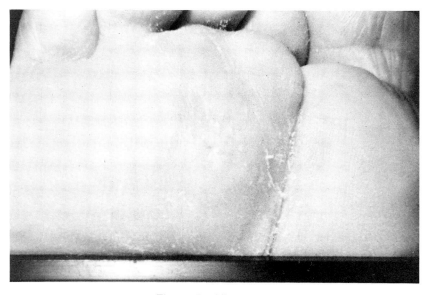

Figure 75. Ulcer healed.

145

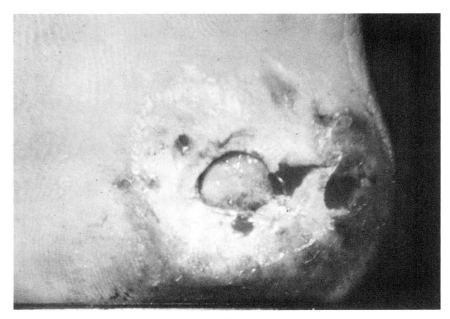

Figure 76. Deep ulceration.

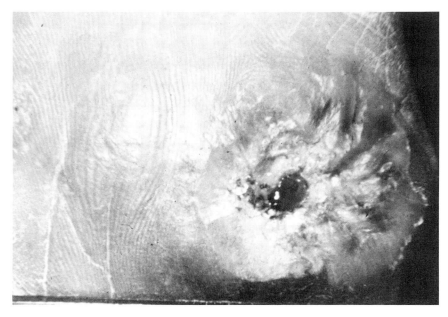

Figure 77. Medial sesamoid excised, same day as Figure 76.

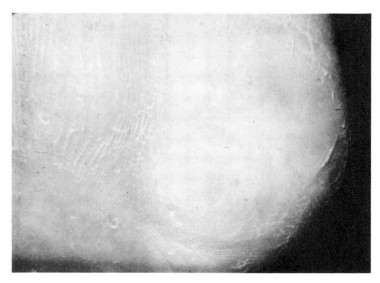

Figure 78. Ulcer healed after seven weeks of therapy involving (1) 4 grams ampicillin daily in divided doses by mouth, (2) instillation of nascent iodine, and (3) bed rest.

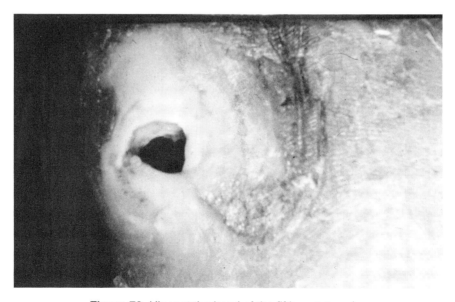

Figure 79. Ulcer at the head of the fifth metatarsal.

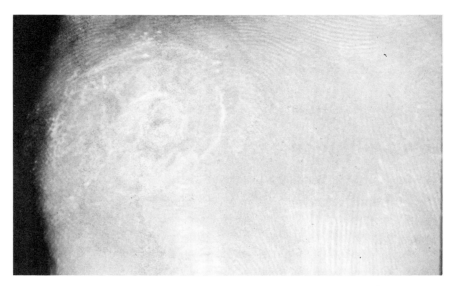

Figure 80. Ulcer healed after eight weeks of treatment including (1) bed rest, (2) excision of metatarsal head, (3) irrigation with nascent iodine solution, and (4) Keflex® 500 mg every 4 hours by mouth.

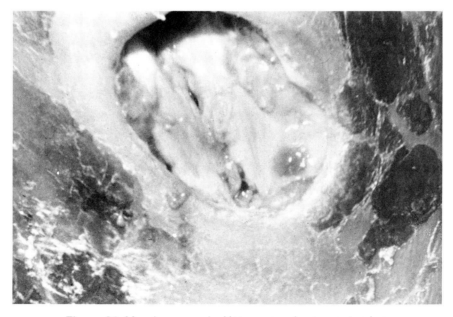

Figure 81. Massive necrosis. Note exposed extensor tendons.

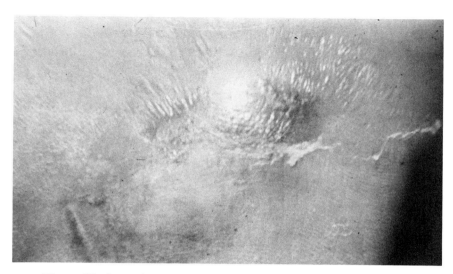

Figure 82. Same foot healed. Treatment included (1) hospitalization (complete bed rest), (2) amikacin 2 grams daily intravenously for 5 days, (3) amoxicillin 2 grams in divided doses daily, (4) tenectomies of exposed extensor tendons, and (5) nascent iodine solution applied daily.

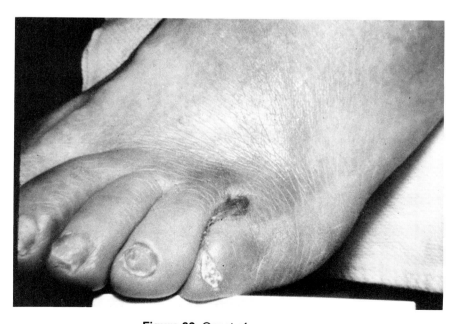

Figure 83. Onset of gangrene.

149

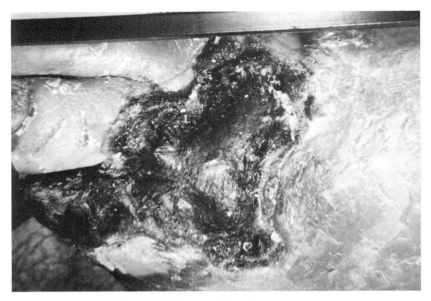

Figure 84. Dry, well-localized gangrene.

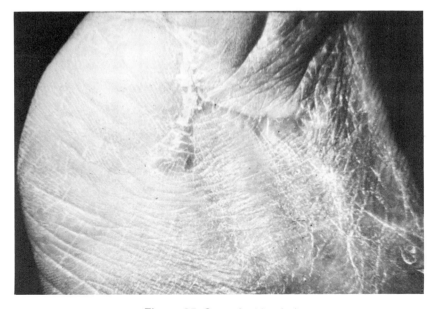

Figure 85. Same foot healed.

Case 9

The patient is a seventy-three year old diabetic male. In addition to having had diabetes for forty years, he has had chronic myelogenous leukemia for four years. His arterial supply is extremely poor. Figure 87 was taken one year after Figure 86. Due to the patient's extremely poor physical condition, it was felt that amputation was contraindicated. It was felt that if sepsis could be avoided, perhaps the limb and the patient's life could be saved. Figure 87 is the reward.

Case 10

The patient is a fifty-five year old male diabetic having had diabetes for ten years. He is presently taking oral hypoglycemic agents for the control of his diabetes. His pedal pulses are present; however, they are of poor quality. The skin temperature and color are normal. As the photographs depict, he has had lesions of his left second, third and fourth toes (Figure 88). The head of the proximal phalanx of the second toe is in the field. No anesthesia was necessary to excise the bone (Figure 89) due to the presence of diabetic neuropathy. The podiatric management of the entire case is given within the text. Figure 90 was taken the same day as Figure 88. Figure 91 was taken one year later.

Case 11

A fifty-five year old male, with a painful lesion of his right great toe, denied having traumatized the affected area.
Past history: He had been a known diabetic for ten years, maintained on 30 units of protamine zinc insulin per day before breakfast. Normo tensive (130/80).
Physical findings: Examination showed a necrotic lesion, secondarily infected. Both the dorsalis pedis and posterior tibial arteries could not be palpated in either foot. Oscillometric readings were as follows: below knee, right:1, left:1½; above ankle, right:trace, left:½.
Laboratory findings: Bacterial culture of the lesion revealed the presence of Proteus. Antibiotic sensitivity studies showed ampicillin to be the drug of choice. His blood count was normal with a normal

differential. Urine examination revealed 1% glucose, negative for albumin.

Diagnosis: This case is an example of a spontaneous infarction of the medial aspect of the right great toe (Figure 92).

Course in hospital: He was treated with 500 mg of ampicillin every four hours by mouth. The lesion was irrigated with the tri-iodide solution daily for two weeks. The white blood cell differential was unaffected. The patient was discharged as healed two months after coming under care (Figure 93).

Case 12

The patient is a fifty-five year old female. She has been a known diabetic for twenty years. During a period of hospitalization for a fractured hip, she developed a decubitus ulcer on the heel of the contralateral limb. This case points out the need for close observation of the feet of those patients who are confined to bed. The heel, as well as any bony prominence, must be protected from decubitus ulcers (Figure 94). Treatment consisted of daily irrigations of the ulcer with a weak iodine solution and appropriate dressing in the form of a doughnut to remove any weight-bearing on the affected area. Culture and sensitivity studies were done every two weeks and the appropriate antibiotic, tetracycline, was given by mouth 500 mg q6h. Figure 95 shows the foot healed.

Case 13

The patient is a forty year old male. He is a known diabetic and has been maintained on a diabetic diet supplemented with two diabinese per day. He is a counterman and, as such, stands throughout his working day. He presented himself for treatment for a lesion on the plantar aspect of the hallux of the left foot; duration of the lesion, three months. X-ray (Figure 96) shows minimal bone destruction and a branch of the princeps hallucis artery is visualized. Culture and sensitivity studies taken every ten days dictated the appropriate antibiotic. He received local debridement and instillation of a weak iodine solution into the slough every week. Figure 97 shows the necrotic periphery and hyperkeratotic perimeter. The proximal phalanx can be seen in the base of the lesion. Figure 98 clearly shows the healed lesion. The patient has been fitted with a latex device to remove weight-bearing during the period required to heal the ulcer.

Case 14

The patient in Figures 99 through 102 show a fifty-five year old, obese diabetic, poorly controlled by insulin and diet. There is a gangrenous lesion at the head of the first metatarsal, medial aspect. Cultural and sensitivity studies were done at the initial visit and massive doses of the appropriate antibiotic were given by mouth. Figure 100 shows a drain in place, saturated with nascent iodine solution. The drain is changed every third day. After debridement (Figure 101) a through and through iodoform drain was inserted. Note the insertion of the hemostat, which transfers the drain into place. Figure 102 shows the patient healed after five months of care which included bed rest, appropriate antibiotics, adequate drainage, debridement as necessary, and control of his diabetes.

Case 15

The patient is a sixty-six year old male diabetic with a lesion at the head of the fifth metatarsal and dorsum of the foot (right foot). Lesion has been present for two months before coming to treatment. Patient was hospitalized immediately, culture and sensitivity studies were done, debridement, lesion was irrigated with nascent iodine solution. Iodoform through and through drain inserted (Figures 103 and 104).

Course in hospital: Work-up consisting of SMA 12, electrolytes, electrocardiogram, chest X-ray, X-ray of both feet, complete blood count and differential, and urinalysis, revealed the following. Blood glucose 210 mg%, electrocardiogram showed evidence of an old mycocardial infarction, X-ray of right foot was not definitive for osteomyelitis at the heads of the second, third and fifth metatarsal bones. Diabetes was controlled by internist employing 25 units protamine insulin daily before breakfast, diabetic (1500 calories) diet. Patient was found to be mildly hypertensive, needing no therapy. Consultation with vascular surgeon carried out. His recommendation was wide incisions and, if they failed, below-knee amputation of right leg. After consultation with patient's family the decision to attempt conservative management was agreed upon. Figures 103 through 113 depict clinical progress.

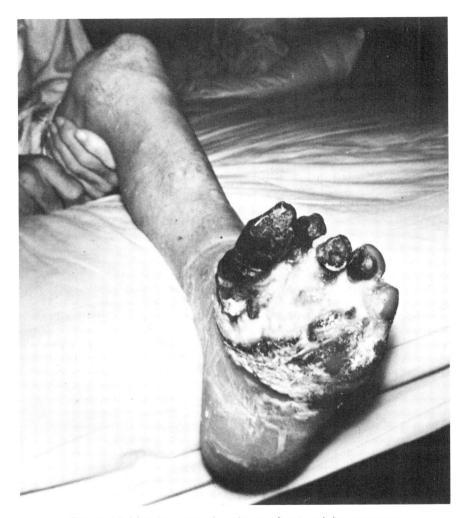

Figure 86. Massive necrosis, mixture of wet and dry gangrene.

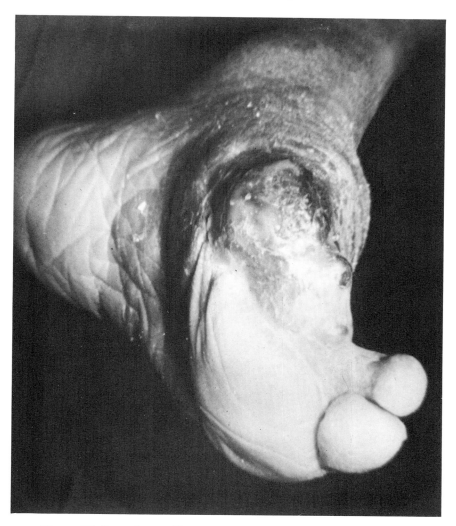

Figure 87. Same foot as Figure 86, healed after one year of treatment including (1) complete bed rest, (2) tetracycline 500 mg 4 times daily for first 3 months, (3) Keflex® 500 mg every 4 hours for 3 months, and (4) nascent iodine dressings throughout treatment.

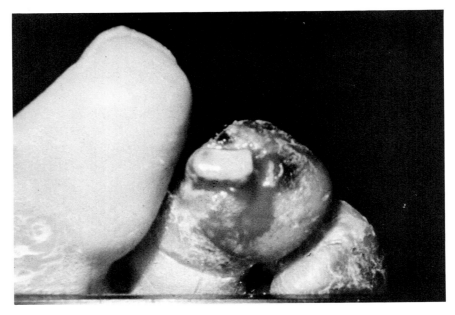

Figure 88. Head of proximal phalanx exposed.

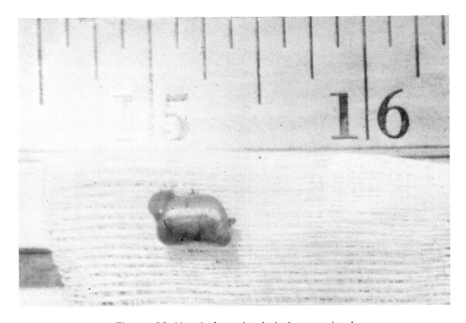

Figure 89. Head of proximal phalanx excised.

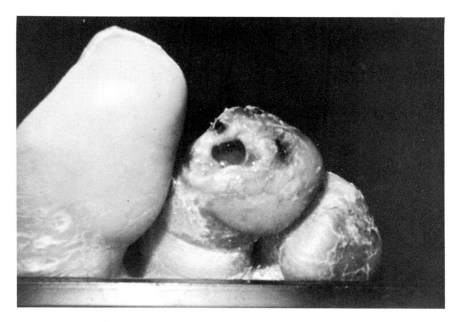

Figure 90. Toe after excision of proximal phalanx.

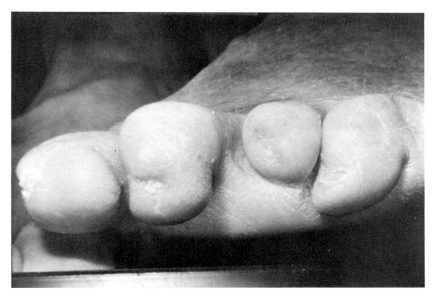

Figure 91. Same toe healed. Treatment included (1) bed rest at home, (2) appropriate antibiotic orally, and (3) nascent iodine packs locally.

157

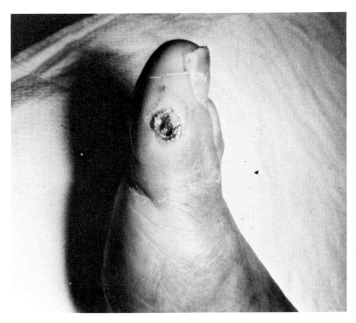

Figure 92. Gangrenous patch on medial aspect of toe, with spontaneous infarction.

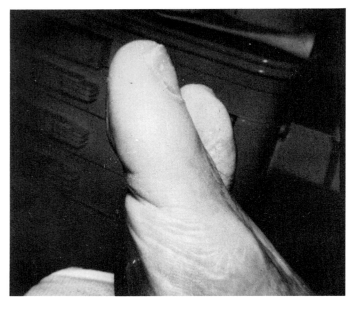

Figure 93. Same toe as Figure 92, healed.

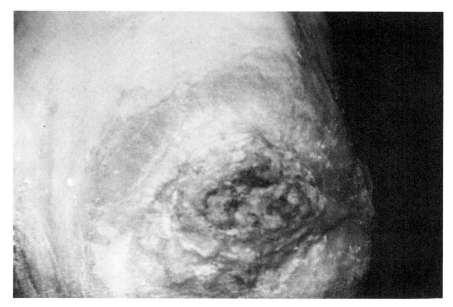

Figure 94. Decubitus ulcer of the heel.

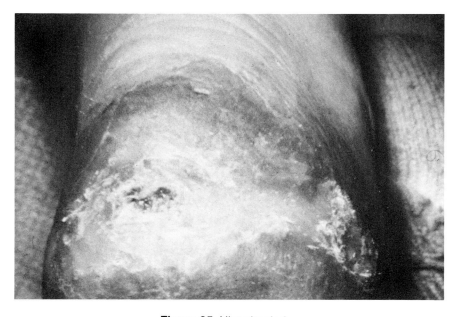

Figure 95. Ulcer healed.

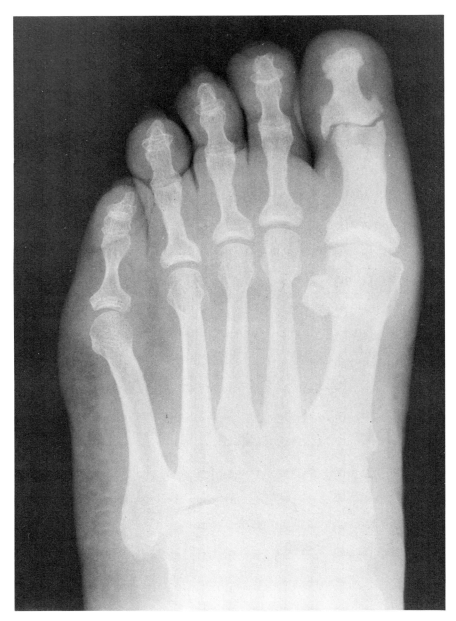

Figure 96. Arteriosclerosis in diabetes. Note calcified princeps hallucis artery.

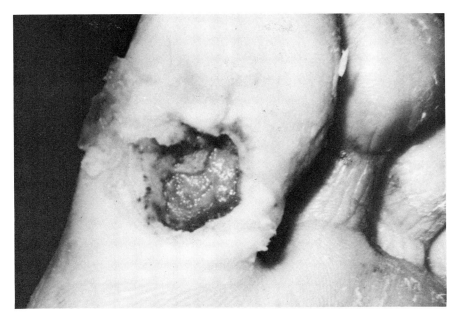

Figure 97. Proximal phalanx visible at base of lesion.

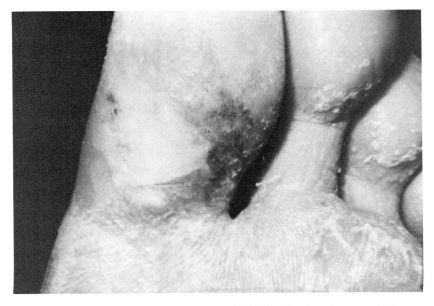

Figure 98. Lesion healed. Treatment included bed rest, appropriate antibiotic and nascent iodine packs.

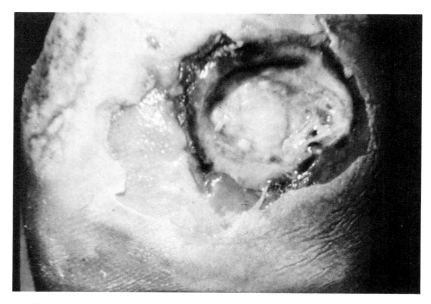

Figure 99. Necrotic ulcer: slough in base, no evidence of granulation tissue.

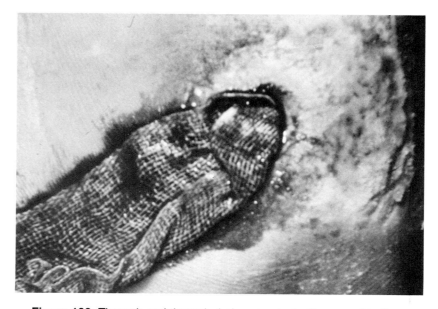

Figure 100. Through and through drain saturated with nascent iodine solution.

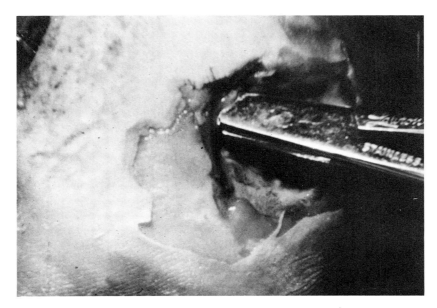

Figure 101. Placing of through and through drain — use of hemostat.

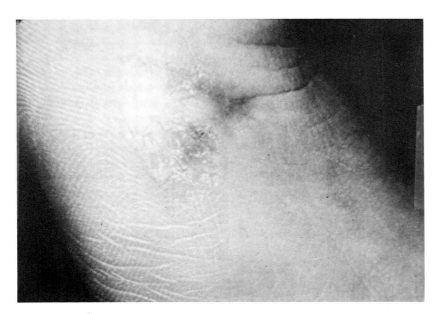

Figure 102. Ulcer healed. Treatment included bed rest, debridement, drain, antibiotic therapy, and nascent iodine irrigation every other day.

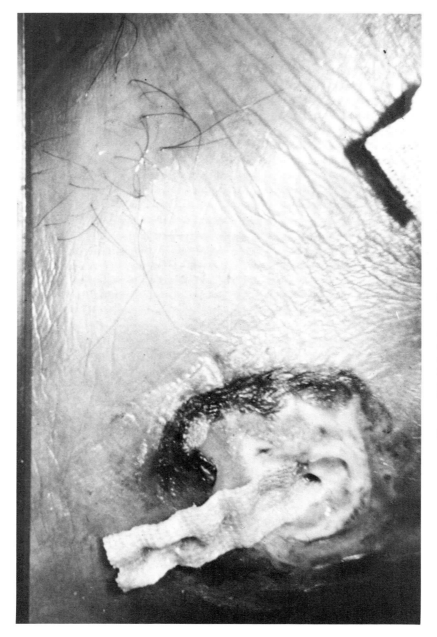

Figure 103. Note hair growth and necrotic ulcer.

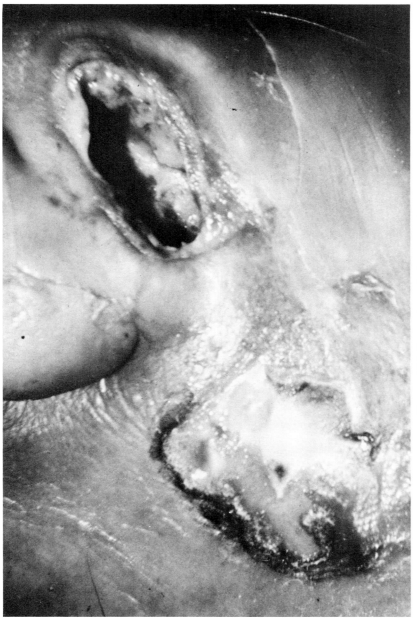

Figure 104. Deep ulcers that communicate.

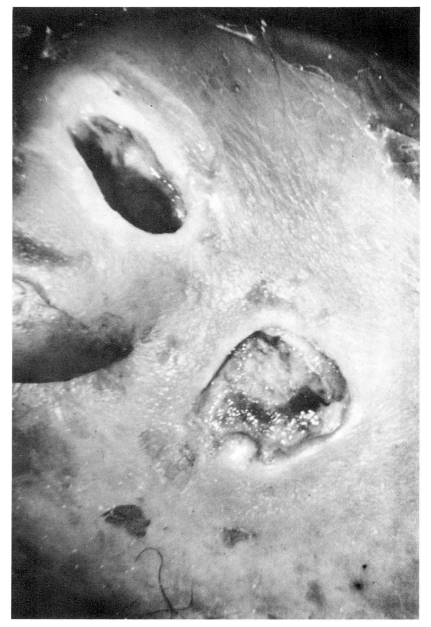

Figure 105. Same foot three weeks later.

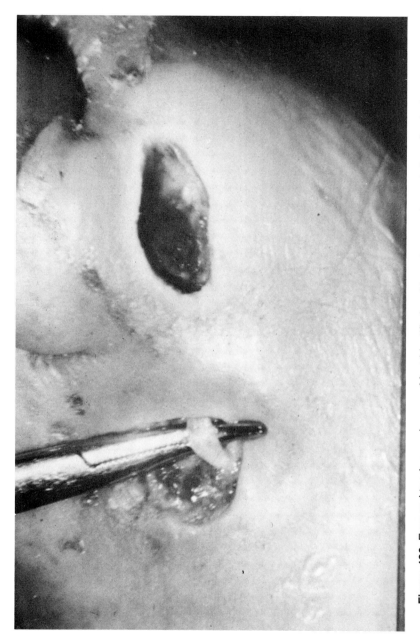

Figure 106. Exposed tendon on dorsum of foot identified and tenectomy performed. A tendon in the base of a lesion will not permit granulation tissue to form and acts as a foreign body.

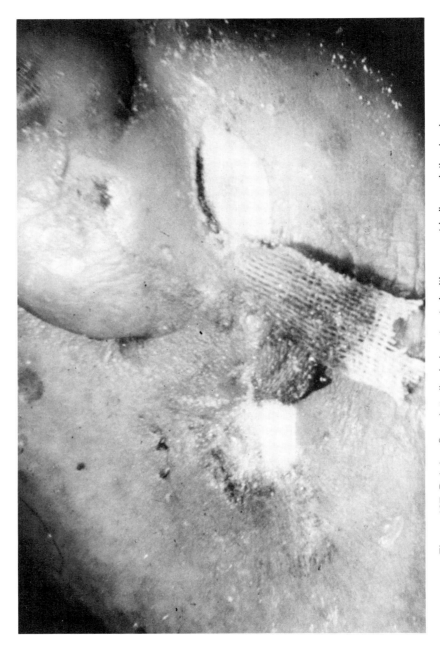

Figure 107. Debrisan® and sterile drain saturated with nascent iodine solution in place.

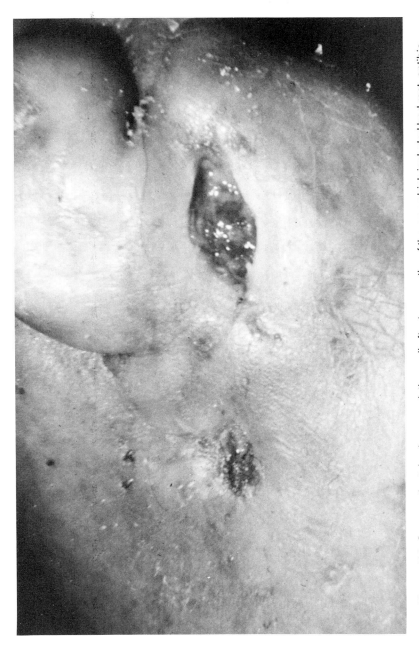

Figure 108. Same patient. Lesion granulating well after two months of therapy which included bed rest, antibiotics, debridement, tenectomy, nascent iodine and Debrisan® crystals.

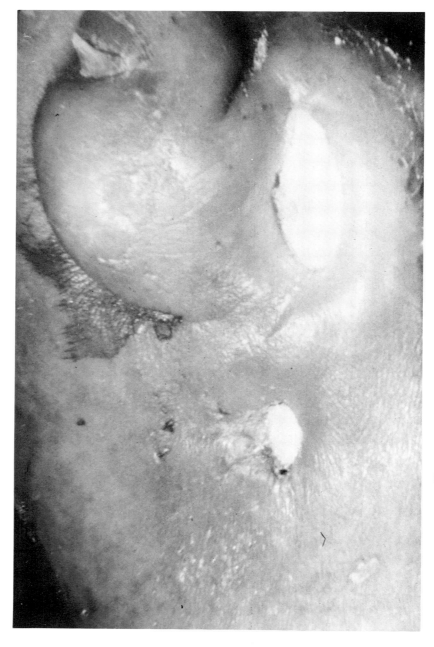

Figure 109. Same patient. Debrisan® crystals placed in lesion.

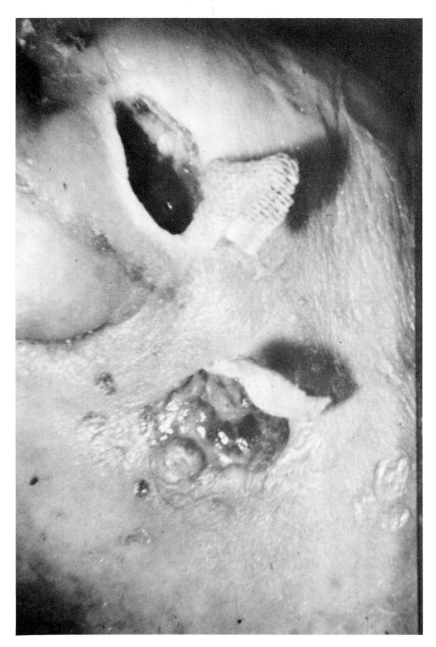

Figure 110. Same patient. Through and through drain in place eleven weeks after treatment.

171

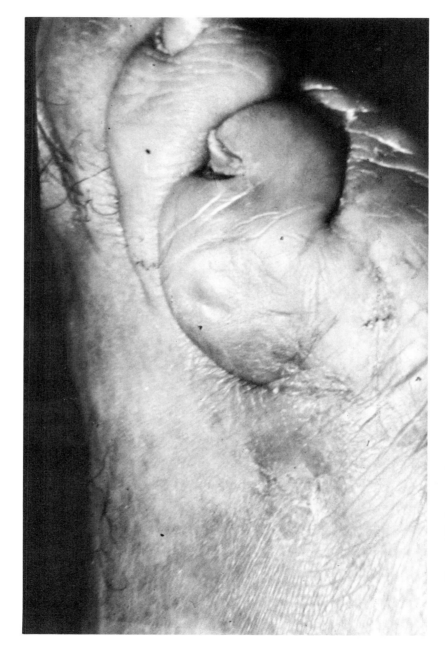

Figure 111. Same patient. Five months after therapy, lesion and sinus tract are completely healed.

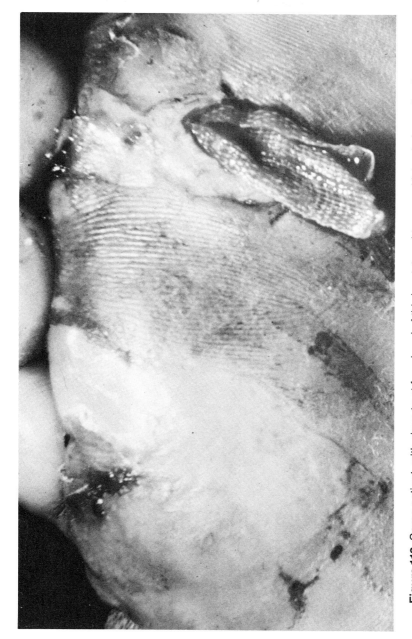

Figure 112. Same patient, with sinus tract from head of third metatarsal to second interphalangeal web space. Treatment was carried out at the same time as that for the lesion at the head of the fifth metatarsal. Note sterile gauze pad saturated with nascent iodine solution in place.

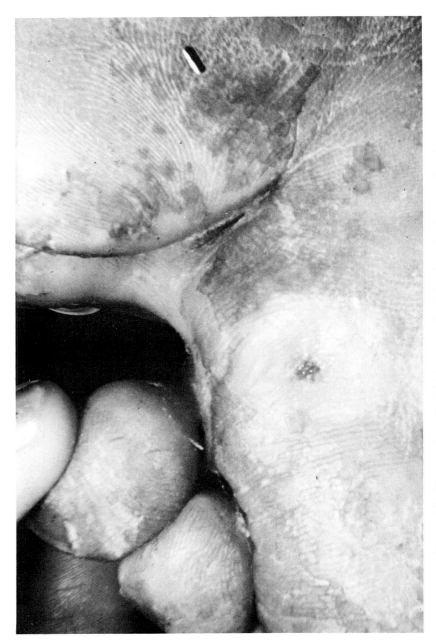

Figure 113. Same patient. Both lesions completely healed after five months of care.

CHAPTER 14

Radiography

Radiography, as we know it today, is a most useful diagnostic aid. The podiatrist must be skilled in the application and interpretation of X-rays. It is not the purpose of this text to teach radiology. I would like to point out the limitations of, as well as the need for, the speciality of radiology within the practice of podiatry.

In previous chapters I have referred to the use of the arteriogram. By the introduction of a radio-opaque material such as Hypaque into the femoral artery and the prompt use of the X-ray apparatus, the radiologist can visualize, for the clinician, exactly the level of obstruction in the arterial pathways. The vascular surgeon can be guided by this procedure and plan possible reconstruction of the arterial system. The limb that is beyond redemption, signified by a poor "run-off" or no "run-off", can be classified by the arteriography.

Atherosclerosis can be visualized in the foot. The diabetic is a candidate for premature arteriosclerosis. It is not uncommon to take an X-ray of a diabetic ulcer, attempting to ascertain the presence of osteomyelitis or neuropathic changes within the osseous structures, and by serendipity find sclerotic vessels.

The ordinary application of the X-ray will show evidence of osteoporosis. Osteoporosis can be visualized on the radiogram and the calcium and phosphorous levels of the blood may be within the normal range. It is not uncommon to find pathologic fractures in the diabetic foot. Every diabetic foot with edema (unilateral) should be X-rayed. All too often the diabetic without any history of trauma will show a fracture of a bone.

The controversy of osteomyelitis versus Charcot's foot may be cleared up with the use of tomography. The radiologist, by means of this radiographic tool, can take X-rays at various levels within a bone. It is possible for the head of a metatarsal, or the shaft of a metatarsal or a tarsal bone, to be visualized at varying depths. Lytic changes can be detected, if present, before overt osteomyelitis is detected.

With the advent of nuclear medicine, the dawn of a new area of investigation is upon us. Diagnosis, therapeutic evaluation, clinical course and prognosis can now be more accurately monitored. The field of bone scans or bone imaging with nuclear material is a complex one and must be left in the hands of those specially trained and certified. The materials used are prepared by skilled technicians and the rectilinear scanner or gamma camera is operated by a board certified nuclear medicine physician. There are several preparations of nuclear material used. They are Osteoscan® (Proctor Gamble) and Technescan® (Mallinckrodt). The former contains 5.9 mg ethane-1 hydroxy-1, 1-diphosphonate and 0.16 mg of stannous chloride. The latter product contains the equivalent of 2.1 mg of the stannous ion and 13.3 mg of pyrophosphate. One milliliter or 15 mCi (millicuries) is slowly injected intraveneously. The material must be injected within three hours of its preparation or its activity is greatly reduced and the results, therefore, are not valid. Patients must be well hydrated before and after the administration of the radioactive material. The patient is encouraged to void as frequently as possible after the injection. This reduces the risk of radiation. Fifty percent of the radioactive material will be excreted in the urine in three hours. Approximately 45-50% is taken up by the bone structure of the body. Four to six percent remains in the blood stream for three hours.

It is important to realize that bone scans may be negative in the early stages of osteomyelitis. More important is the fact that in the presence of arterial impairment or basement membrane disease, as we so commonly find in the diabetic foot, the bone scan can be negative for early osteomyelitis. A positive scan, on the other hand, will confirm the presence of clinically suspected osteomyelitis. A positive bone scan for osteomyelitis can be obtained four to six weeks after appropriate and satisfactory treatment. One may obtain a positive bone scan in the healing phase of osteomyelitis. Alazraki et al[1] report that using Gallium and Tc[99m] phosphate increases the sensitivity and specificity of the scintigraphy for osteomyelitis.

RADIOGRAPHY

Ten minutes after the injection of polymer of phosphorous (1 ml or 15 mCi) the osteomyelitic area will appear bright red on the scan using a gamma camera. The technique is advanced and sophisticated, with the final scan recorded on a tape cassette.

REFERENCE

1. Alazraki, N.P., Fierer, J., and Resnick, D.: The role of gallium and bone scanning in monitoring response to therapy in chronic osteomyelitis. *J. Nuclear Med.*, **19**:696, 1978.

CHAPTER 15

Notes and Observations

Culture and sensitivity studies are not the final and ultimate criteria for antibiotic therapy. Clinical judgment and minute management are vital.

The use of antibiotics can be overemphasized. The use of antibiotics should be reserved only for an infectious process. It is poor clinical management to overload the patient with antibiotics if the cardinal signs of infection are not present. Do not be lulled into a sense of false security by prescribing a "broad-spectrum" antibiotic for the treatment of a denuded area occurring on the diabetic foot. It is much wiser and safer to apply a local antiseptic and antibiotic dressing to a denuded area than to prescribe large doses of an oral or parenteral antibiotic immediately. Antibiotics are potent and may have serious side effects. They should be used only when clinical judgment dictates, after weighing the "pros" and "cons".

Thickening of the basement membrane of the capillaries plays an important role in the increased susceptibility of diabetics to infections.[1] Increase in width of the muscular layer of the capillaries in the diabetic is greatest in the lower extremity.[2] The foot is most susceptible to infections resulting in gangrene. This can and does occur in spite of the presence of pedal pulses.

Diabetes mellitus is a disease which adversely effects the blood flow to the foot and toes. Literature to date seems to make it clear that despite exquisite control of the glucose level of the blood, the complications of diabetes (vascular disease, retinopathy, neuropathy and nephropathy) occur with some frequency in the poorly controlled diabetic.

Complete avoidance of weight-bearing is necessary to heal ulcers occurring on the foot. The podiatrist can treat the patient with the proper antibiotics or combination of antibiotics. He may use triple iodine solution, Debrisan® and local antibiotics and fail. The physician can control the diabetes and levels of cholesterol, and still the patient will lose his leg. The key therapeutic strategy is total bed rest.

Plasma lipoproteins — cholesterol, triglycerides and phospholipids — have not in themselves proven the sole etiological factors in arteriosclerosis. Exogenous hyperlipema cannot be indicted for sclerotic vessels. I believe there are enzyme systems, yet to be discovered, which are the etiological basis for arteriosclerosis and arteriosclerotic degeneration. The pathogenesis of vascular occlusive disease has yet to be unraveled. This is true for the diabetic as well as the non-diabetic. All we have today is statistical evidence of an acceleration in the development of vascular disease in the diabetic.

So-called vascular exercises (Buerger's exercises) can be detrimental. During the phase of leg elevation, one is placing a further restriction on an already compromised blood flow.

Vasodilators have no place in the management of occlusive, organic vascular disease of the feet and legs. In spite of sympathectomy and autosympathectomy, gangrene occurs and limbs are lost.

Whitehouse et al[3] state that a diabetic amputee has a greater likelihood of losing his life from a complication of diabetes than of losing his remaining limb. Two-thirds (66%) of the diabetics who lose a limb due to arterial impairment will not live more than five years.[4]

Amputation of a gangrenous toe by the surgeon in the absence of pedal pulses is the first procedure, followed closely by mid-foot, then below or above knee amputation. Arteriography and arterial reconstruction, when feasible, is the logical surgical approach prior to amputation of a toe.

Root[5] has reported that 66% of diabetics with open lesion have amputations of the toe, foot or limb. Schalt[6] reports an amputation rate of 52% in diabetics with open lesions. Collens and Rakow[7] report a low amputation rate of 11% in a series of cases of gangrenous lesions of the foot and/or toes in the diabetic. Warren et al[8] report 29% of diabetics have gangrene or amputation of an extremity. If the rate of amputation is to decrease, the hospital must furnish competent podiatric services in both the out-patient and in-patient areas of the hospital. In 1950, Bell[9] reported that among patients with arterial impairment, gangrene is forty times more common in the diabetic than in the non-diabetic.

Gangrene can be iatrogenically induced. If the examining physician or podiatrist is pressing his finger against the foot with sufficient pressure to blanch his own nail bed, the result is all too often frank gangrene in a vascular deficient foot.

Clinically and roentgonographically, it is very difficult to distinguish between osteomyelitis and osseous lesions in the diabetic who has peripheral neuropathy.[10]

In 1970, Ecker[11] reported a 61% survival rate three years after amputation.

Over 40% of unilateral leg amputations will require some form of amputations on the remaining limb within five years.

Patients are poor historians (to phrase it politely). When gangrene occurs, all they remember is a visit to a podiatrist for nail cutting or a similar minor procedure. They conveniently forget such things as the use of a razor on the callus by the patient, who, incidently, is half blind due to retinopathy, or the hot bath — due to his neuropathy, he cannot distinguish hot and cold, let alone degrees of temperature — or they cannot recall striking a foot against a chair. The same arteriosclerosis that distorts the patient's memory and vision has caused the necrosis of his toe. It has proven financially convenient to try to blame the podiatrist. I am always amazed by the appearance of children and other parasitic relatives when they think some money can be made by starting a malpractice action.

Acute infarction with resulting gangrene occurs spontaneously in the feet of the diabetic and the non-diabetic.[12] The etiology and the pathogeneis of myocardial or cerebral infarction are similar — namely, arteriosclerosis. The cardiologist or the internist is never blamed for these "acts of God". The foot is part of the body just as the vital organs are. Why is the foot exempt from "acts of God"?

REFERENCES

1. Banson, B.B., and Lacy, P.E.: Diabetic microangiopathy in human toes, with emphasis on the ultrastructural change in dermal capillaries. *Am. J. Pathol.* **45**:41, 1964.

2. Williamson, J.R., Vogler, N.J., and Kilo, C.: Microvascular disease in diabetes. *Med. Clin. North Am.*, **55**:847, 1971.

3. Whitehouse, F.W., Jurgenson, C., and Block, M.A.: The later life of the diabetic amputee. *Diabetes*, **17**:520, 1968.

4. Levin, M.E. and O'Neal, L.W.: *The Diabetic Foot*, C.V. Mosby St. Louis, 1977.

5. Root, H.F.: Collected study of nine hospitals in Boston area. *New Eng. J. Med.*, **253**:685, 1955.

6. Schalt, D.C.: Chronic arteriosclerotic occlusion of femoral artery. *J.A.M.A.*, **175**:937, 1961.

7. Collens, W.S., and Rakow, R.B.: Conservative management of gangrene in the diabetic. *J.A.M.A.*, **181**:692, 1962.

8. Warren, S., Le Conpte, P.M., and Legg, M.A.: *Pathology of Diabetes*, Lea and Febiger, Philadelphia, 1966.

9. Bell, E.T.: Incidence of gangrene of the extremities in non-diabetic and in diabetic persons. *Arch. Pathol.*, **28**:27, 1969.

10. Friedmen, S.A., and Rakow, R.B.: Osseous lesions of the foot in diabetic neuropathy. *Diabetes*, **20**:302, 1971.

11. Ecker, L.M., and Jacobs, B.S.: Lower extremity amputation in diabetic patients. *Diabetes*, **19**:189, 1970.

12. Rakow, R.B.: The treatment of necrotic lesions in the diabetic patient. *J.A.P.A.*, **57**:412, 1967.

INDEX

INDEX